An Introduction to Animal Physiology

An Introduction to Animal Physiology

Per Svendsen

MTP
MEDICAL AND TECHNICAL PUBLISHING CO LTD

Published by

MTP

Medical and Technical Publishing Co Ltd
P.O. Box 55
St Leonard's House,
St Leonardgate, Lancaster
Copyright © 1974; Per Svendsen
ISBN 0 852001142 [Cased edition]
ISBN 0 85200049 9 [Limp edition]
First published 1974

PRINTED AND BOUND IN GREAT BRITAIN BY
EYRE & SPOTTISWOODE LTD
THANET PRESS, MARGATE

ALTHOUGH PHYSIOLOGY IS INCREASINGLY IMPORTANT IN the study of agriculture there are no physiology texts written specifically for agricultural students. This one has therefore been produced to prepare the student for the study of animal nutrition and animal production. Special emphasis has been given to the physiology of digestion and reproduction in domestic animals. It is my hope that the book may also be useful in the training of animal health assistants and as an introductory text in physiology for students of veterinary science.

The manuscript was reviewed by Professor D. Robertshaw, Dr. P. S. Bramley and Dr. D. F. Horrobin and typed by Mrs. F. Hansford. I wish to express my thanks for their valuable contributions.

I would furthermore like to express my gratitude to Dr. D. F. Horrobin for allowing me to use illustrations from his books, *Medical Physiology and Biochemistry*, published by Edward Arnold, *Essential Biochemistry, Endocrinology and Nutrition*, and *Essential Physiology*, published by MTP Ltd., and to Professor Johs Moustgaard for permission to reproduce tables from his book, *Husdyrenes Fysiologi og Etnæringsfysiologi*.

PER SVENDSEN,
Nairobi, Kenya

Contents

1

Homeostasis and control systems

CELLULAR STRUCTURE AND FUNCTION

The membrane which surrounds the cell is a remarkable structure. It is not only semipermeable, allowing some structures to pass through it and excluding others, but its permeability can be varied. It is generally referred to as the unit or plasma membrane, and despite differences in functional characteristics its basic structure seems to be the same throughout the whole animal and plant kingdom. The unit membrane is also found surrounding the organelles inside the cell.

The unit membrane is approximately 75 Å thick. It is made up of an inner 20 Å layer of protein, a middle 35 Å layer of lipid, and an outer 20 Å layer of protein and polysaccharide. The membrane behaves as if it contained holes or pores 3 Å in diameter. These pores allow small molecules to pass the membrane, whereas larger molecules pass through the membrane by becoming dissolved in it, or by some other process.

The nucleus is present in all cells that divide. It is made up in large part of the chromosomes, the structures that carry the heritable characteristics of the animal. During cell division, the pairs of chromosomes become visible. Each chromosome is made up of supporting protein and a giant molecule of deoxyribonucleic acid (DNA). The ultimate units of heredity are the genes on the chromosomes, and each gene is a portion of the DNA molecule.

During normal cell division by mitosis, the chromosomes duplicate themselves and then divide in such a way that each daughter cell receives a full number of chromosomes. During their final maturation, germ cells undergo a division in which the chromosomes do not duplicate themselves, and half of them go to each daughter cell. As a result of this meiosis, mature spermatozoa and ova contain only half the normal number of chromosomes. When spermatozoa and ova unite, the resultant cell has a full complement of chromosomes.

The mitochondria are oval-shaped structures containing enzymes concerned with the electron transfers responsible for the synthesis of the high-energy phosphate compound adenosine triphosphate (ATP). This molecule is the principle energy source for energy-requiring reactions in animals and plants. The enzymes on the outside of the mitochondria are mainly concerned with biological oxidations, providing raw material for the citric acid cycle inside the mitochondria. The mitochondria are thus the power-generating units of the cell, and are most plentiful in parts of cells where energy requiring processes take place.

In the cytoplasm of the cell, there are large, somewhat irregular structures surrounded by unit membrane. These organelles are the lysosomes. They contain a variety of enzymes believed to function as a form of digestive system for the cell. Exogenous substances, such as bacteria, which become engulfed by the cell, end up in a vacuole where they mix with the contents of a lysosome. Some of the products of this process are absorbed into the cytoplasm, whereas the rest are removed from the cell by rupture of the vacuole to the exterior of the cell.

Other structures in the cell are the centrioles which are concerned with the movements of chromosomes during cell division, and the Golgi complex which has a secretory function.

Chemical composition of the cell

About 85 per cent of the cell is water which occurs either as free water or absorbed to the surface of protein molecules. Water is formed by oxidation of hydrogen during metabolism and removed by excretion via skin, lungs, kidneys, and intestine. Since water is excreted faster than it is formed, additional water must be taken from outside. The quantity varies with the environment and the turnover rate of water in the animal. About 10 per cent of the cell is protein. It functions as enzymes and as structural matter, and it maintains the colloid osmotic pressure. Lipids are mainly found in the cell membrane and account for only 2 per cent of the cell. Carbohydrates are found in combination with nucleic acid to form deoxyribonucleic acid and ribonucleic acid. Carbohydrates make up about 1·5 per cent of the cell. Inorganic substances, 1·5 per cent of the cell, aid in maintaining a constant pH and regulate the osmotic pressure within the cell.

The materials found in the cell cytoplasm are largely in a colloidal solution. The colloidal particles range in diameter from 1 to 500 mμ. and do not pass selectively permeable membranes.

Body fluid compartments

The cells of the body exist in an 'internal sea' of extracellular fluid. From this fluid the cells take up oxygen and nutrients, and into it they discharge metabolic waste products. The extracellular fluid is divided into two components, the interstitial fluid and the circulating blood plasma. The plasma and the cellular elements of the blood fill the vascular system, and together they form the total blood volume.

The volume of the body fluid compartments can be measured by injection of a known amount of a substance which will distribute itself evenly and completely throughout the compartment to be measured, e.g. the plasma compartment or the extracellular compartment. After a mixing period a sample of the fluid is drawn and the concentration of the substance determined. The volume can then be calculated in the following way:

$$\text{Volume} = \frac{\text{amount}}{\text{concentration}}$$

Plasma volume has been measured by using dyes which become bound in plasma proteins, particularly Evans's blue. The extracellular fluid volume is difficult to measure because the limits of this space are ill defined and because few substances mix rapidly enough in all parts of the compartment to remain exclusively extracellular. The most accurate measurement of the extracellular fluid volume is obtained by using inulin. The intracellular fluid volume cannot be measured directly, but it can be calculated by subtracting the extracellular fluid volume from total body water. Total body water can be measured by the same dilution principle used to measure the other body spaces. Deuterium oxide (heavy water) is most frequently used.

In the adult domestic animal the amount of water is about 70 per cent of the body weight, 50 per cent of the body weight is intracellular fluid, 15 per cent interstitial fluid, and 5 per cent plasma.

Composition of body fluids

The intracellular and extracellular fluid compartments differ in electrolyte composition. The most striking differences are the relatively low concentration of protein anions in the extracellular fluid

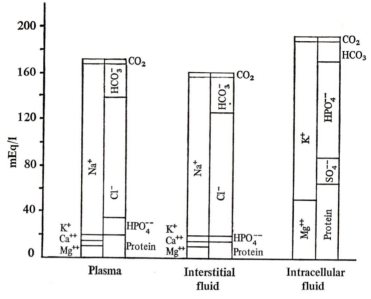

Fig.1.1. The ionic composition of the body fluids (in mEq/1 water).

compared to the intracellular fluid, and the fact that Na^+ and Cl^- are largely extracellular, whereas most of the K^+ is intracellular (Fig. 1.1).

The differences in composition of the various body fluid compartments are due to the nature of the membranes of the cells separating the intracellular and interstitial fluid, and the capillary wall separating the plasma from the interstitial fluid. The forces producing movement of water and small molecules across these barriers are diffusion due to concentration gradients and electrical gradients, differences in osmotic pressure and hydrostatic pressure, differences in membrane permeability, and active transport of certain molecules or ions across the membrane.

Diffusion is the process by which a gas or a substance in solution spreads, because of the motion of its particles. Since the particles (ions or molecules) are in random movement they frequently collide. They therefore tend to move from areas of high concentration to areas of low concentration. Diffusion of ions is also affected by their electrical charges. Whenever there is a difference in potential between two areas, positive ions move down the electrical gradient to the more negatively charged area, negative ions move the opposite way.

The difference in hydrostatic pressure on each side of a biological membrane causes filtration of fluid. The amount of fluid filtered in a given time is proportionate to the difference in pressure and the surface area of the membrane. Molecules which are smaller in diameter than the pores of the membrane pass through with the fluid, whereas larger molecules are retained.

Osmosis is the movement of solvent molecules across a membrane into an area in which there is a higher concentration of a solute to which the membrane is impermeable. The movement can be prevented by applying pressure to the more concentrated solution. The pressure necessary to prevent solvent movement is known as the effective osmotic pressure.

The membrane permeability differs for different particles. The diameter of the particle compared to the diameter of the membrane pore is of importance as well as the solubility of the particle. Fat soluble molecules will be more likely to pass the membrane than water soluble molecules.

Diffusion, filtration, and osmosis are all passive processes in the sense that they require no energy supply. The molecules involved move down concentration or electrical gradients. There are, however, many instances in the body in which ions or molecules are moved against concentration gradients, osmotic pressure, and electrical gradients. Such movement is defined as active transport and requires energy.

The distribution of ions in the body fluid compartments is a result of the combined forces mentioned above. The effect is known as the Donnan equilibrium. When there is an ion on one side of a membrane that cannot diffuse through the membrane, the distribution of the other ions to which the membrane is permeable is affected in a predictable way. If, for example, isotonic solutions of B^+Q^- and A^+P^- are separated by a membrane permeable to A^+, B^+, and Q^-, but not permeable to P^- (Fig.1.2,A), the concentration gradients will tend to move A^+, B^+, and Q^-, whereas P^- will remain on one side owing to its impermeability. Initially A^+ and B^+ movements will cancel out. The movement of Q^-, however, will be halted because P^- cannot move the opposite way. Negative charge will thus build up on the side where P^- is present. When the electrical force keeping Q^- out becomes equal to the concentration gradient pushing it in, net movement of Q^- will cease. There will thus be an excess of P^- and negative charge on the right side of the membrane (Fig.1.2,B). To maintain electroneutrality there must be equal numbers of positive and negative ions on both sides of the membrane. Positive ions must, therefore, move from left to right. Equal numbers of A^+ and B^+ will move. On the left side of the membrane we find that the concentration of A^+ = concentration of B^+ and that the concentration of A^+ + concentration of B^+ = concentration of Q^-. On the right side of the membrane the concentration of A^+ = concentration of B^+, but the concentration of A^+ + concentration of B^+ = concentration of Q^- + concentration of P^-. As a result of this, the total concentration of ions on the right side is larger than the total concentration of ions on the left side. An osmotic pressure gradient has thus been created which tends to move water from the left to the right side.

This demonstrates that when a membrane separates two solutions, one of which contains a non-diffusible ion, the equilibrium becomes unstable. Stability can be achieved by rigid walls, as in plant cells, by hydrostatic forces which oppose the tendency of water to move across the membrane, or by active transport mechanisms which move ions against the electrochemical gradient to maintain the solution isotonic (Fig.1.2,C).

Fluid balance between plasma and tissue

When the blood leaves the heart (Chapter 11) it travels first along the arteries. The arteries break up into smaller vessels known as arterioles and these arterioles give rise to the tiny capillaries. The capillaries then join up to give venules and veins which carry the blood back to the heart. Only the capillaries, which have walls one cell thick, are thin enough to allow rapid exchange of fluid and dissolved material between the blood and the interstitial fluid outside the blood vessels.

The capillary wall is freely permeable to water and all particles below a certain size, but impermeable to colloid particles such as protein molecules. The forces that govern the transport of fluid across the capillary endothelium are primarily differences in hydrostatic pressure and colloid osmotic pressure between the plasma in the capillary and the interstitial fluid surrounding the capillaries. The blood pressure in the capillary represents the hydrostatic pressure. It is considerably higher in the arterial end of the capillary than in the venous end. The difference in colloid osmotic pressure between the plasma and the interstitial fluid is due to the different protein concentrations in the two fluid compartments. The hydrostatic pressure of the interstitial fluid is considerably smaller than that of the plasma.

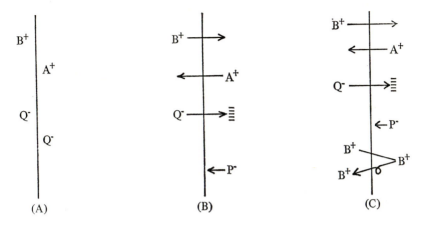

Fig. 1.2.

Fluid will tend to leave the capillary under the combined forces of the capillary blood pressure and the interstitial colloid osmotic pressure. At the same time fluid will enter the capillary under the influence of the colloid osmotic pressure of plasma and the hydrostatic pressure of the interstitial fluid (Fig.1.3).

REGULATION OF ACID-BASE BALANCE

The pH of the extracellular fluid is maintained at 7·4. This value usually varies less than 0·1 pH unit. The pH is stabilized by the buffering capacity of the body fluids. A buffer is a substance which has the ability to bind or release H^+ in solution, thus maintaining the pH of a solution relatively constant despite the addition of considerable quantities of acid or base.

Several buffers are found in the blood, both in the red blood cells and in the plasma. In the cells haemoglobin and oxyhaemoglobin are the major buffers, in the plasma the proteins and the bicarbonate show a large buffering capacity. One buffer, carbonic acid, accounts for more than 50 per cent of the activity. Carbonic acid is normally dissociated into bicarbonate and hydrogen ions:

$$CO_2 + H_2O \rightleftharpoons H_2CO_3 \rightleftharpoons HCO_3^- + H^+$$

Addition of hydrogen ions will cause the equilibrium to shift to the left so that the added hydrogen is removed from the solution.

Removal of hydrogen, on the other hand, will cause the equilibrium
to move to the right and more carbonic acid dissociates. At a certain
hydrogen concentration equal concentrations of carbonic acid and
bicarbonate are found in the solution. This pH is defined as the pK
of the solution.

An acid may be defined as a substance which can give off hydrogen
ions into solution while a base is one which can take up hydrogen
ions from solution. The most important acid-base system in the body
is the one which links carbonic acid and bicarbonate. Carbonic acid
is an acid because it can split up to give hydrogen ions and bicarbonate
ions. Bicarbonate is a base because bicarbonate ions can combine
with hydrogen ions so removing them from solution.

It has been discovered that the relationship between hydrogen
ions, carbonic acid and bicarbonate ions can be expressed by the
following equation:

$$pH = pK + log \frac{[HCO_3^-]}{[H_2CO_3]}$$

pH is a shorthand way of describing the hydrogen ion concentration.
It is in fact the negative logarithm of the hydrogen ion concentration. pH 7 means that the hydrogen ion concentration is 10^{-7}
mEq/l: pH 6 means that it is 10^{-6} mEq/l and so on. The important
things to note are that each unit change in pH means a 10-fold
change in hydrogen ion concentration and that a falling pH means a
rising acidity.

From this equation one can see the meaning of pK. When the
bicarbonate and carbonic acid concentrations are equal (i.e. $[HCO_3^-]$
$= [H_2CO_3]$), then the expression on the far right of the equation
will be log 1. But log 1 = 0 and so pK must then equal pH. The pK
is therefore the pH value at which half of an acid-base system is in
the form of an acid (e.g. H_2CO_3) and half is in the form of a base
(HCO_3^-). For the carbonic acid-bicarbonate system the pK is 6·1.

It has been found that the concentration of carbonic acid is equal
to the partial pressure of carbon dioxide (pCO_2) multiplied by a constant which at normal body temperatures is equal to 0·03. The equation may therefore be rewritten as follows:

$$pH = 6·1 + log \frac{[HCO_3^-]}{0·03\ pCO_2}$$

In this equation there are only three variable factors: the pH, the
bicarbonate ion concentration and the pCO_2. This means that if two

	Arterial end	Venous end
Colloid osmotic pressure	25 mmHg	25 mmHg
Blood pressure	32 mmHg	12 mmHg
Colloidal osmotic pressure	10 mmHg	10 mmHg
Fluid pressure	5 mmHg	5 mmHg
	12 mmHg	8 mmHg

Fig.1.3. Diagram showing the fluid movements across the capillary membrane. In the arterial end fluid leaves the capillary under a pressure of 32 + 10 = 42 mmHg, and enters into the capillary under a pressure of 25 + 5 = 30 mmHg. The net movement thus being from plasma to interstitial fluid under a pressure of 12 mmHg. In the venous end fluid leaves under a pressure of 12 + 10 = 22 mmHg and enters a pressure of 25 + 5 = 30 mmHg, resulting in a net movement from interstitial fluid to plasma under a pressure of 8 mmHg.

of these variables can be fixed by the body, the third will automatically also be fixed. The kidneys maintain constant the bicarbonate concentration of the blood while the respiratory system maintains the pCO_2 constant. The pH is thus automatically regulated by the combined operations of the kidneys and lungs.

From the equation it can be seen that an increase in the bicarbonate concentration will cause a rise in the pH while a rise in the pCO_2 will cause a fall in pH. In order to keep the pH constant, a fall in the bicarbonate concentration must be compensated by a similar fall in the partial pressure of carbon dioxide. This is brought about by an increased repiratory rate (Chapter 12). If on the other hand bicarbonate is added to the blood, the pH will rise. This in turn causes a fall in respiratory rate and the partial pressure of carbon dioxide increases so returning the pH to its normal level.

MAINTENANCE OF THE INTERNAL ENVIRONMENT

The maintenance of the composition of the extracellular fluid is known as homeostasis. Homeostasis is achieved by the combined action of the various organ systems of the body. With the many organ systems involved, an accurate control and coordination is necessary. Such a coordination is carried out by the control systems of the body—the sense organs, the nervous system and the endocrine system.

2

Nervous system

CONTROL MECHANISMS

The general principle of control is to collect as much information as possible about the external surroundings and about what goes on inside the body. This information, which may be conscious or unconscious, is used to direct the activity of muscles and glands. This activity may be voluntary or involuntary. Two systems of the body, the nervous system and the endocrine system, are concerned with the communications within the animal body.

The nervous system consists of separate cells, the neurons. A typical spinal motor neuron consists of a cell body with an elongated nerve fibre, the axon, projecting from it. The cell body has numerous short projections known as dendrites. Axons from other neurons make contact with the dendrites, but there is always a minute gap between one neuron and the next. The region of contact between two neurons is known as a synapse. The nerve impulses are initiated in the cell body and travel outwards along the axon. The nerve cells act on other neurons by releasing small amounts of a chemical known as transmitter substance into the synapse. The chemical then initiates another impulse in the next neuron. If the neuron makes contact with a muscle fibre or a gland cell, the chemical will cause either contraction or secretion. The chemical released by the synapse is rapidly destroyed by a special enzyme to prevent its action from being too prolonged.

The endocrine system like the nervous system releases chemicals, hormones, which are carried by the blood to every cell in the animal body. Some hormones, for instance the thyroid hormone act on all cells. Others like the sex hormones have a more marked effect on special tissues, the target organs. A further stage of specificity is shown by some of the hormones released by the pituitary glands. The thyroid stimulating hormone is released into the blood and carried to every cell in the body. However, it acts only on cells of the

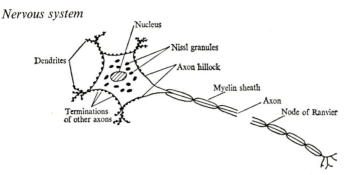

Fig.2.1. A typical motor neuron (from Horrobin, *Medical Physiology and Biochemistry*, by kind permission of the author and Edward Arnold, 1968).

thyroid gland, stimulating them to produce the thyroid hormone. The adrenocorticotrophic hormone acts only on the adrenal cortex and the gonadotrophins act only on the sex glands.

Just as the pituitary gland controls other endocrine glands, it is itself under the control of the brain. The gland is connected by a stalk to the part of the brain known as the hypothalamus. Blood which has passed through the hypothalamus flows down the pituitary stalk and into the capillaries of the gland. Nerve cells in the hypothalamus release chemicals into the blood. These are carried to the pituitary where they act on the cells to control the production of the hormones. These chemicals or releasing factors are not true hormones in that they are not released into the blood as a whole. They are rather to be recognized as a graduation between a hormone and a nervous transmitter.

There is thus no sharp distinction between the nervous system and the endocrine system. They are both control mechanisms which involve interaction between cells.

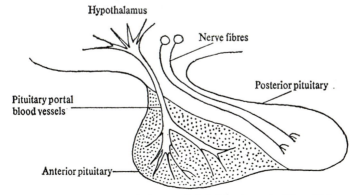

Fig.2.2. The hypothalamus, pituitary and their blood supply (Horrobin).

THE REFLEX ARC

The afferent or incoming parts of the nervous system are linked to the efferent or outgoing motor parts. When a piece of sensory information produces a response which is not voluntarily controlled, the sequence of events is said to be a reflex. The basic unit of this integrated activity is the reflex arc (Fig.2.3). The arc consists of a sense organ, an afferent neuron, one or more synapses in a central integrating section, an efferent neuron, and an effector. In mammals the connection between afferent and efferent somatic neurons is in the brain or spinal cord. The afferent neurons enter via the dorsal roots of the spinal cord or the cranial nerves of the brain. The efferent fibres leave via the ventral roots or corresponding motor cranial nerves. The reflex arc is frequently extended by the action of a hormone. For example, stimulation of the teats reflexly causes the posterior lobe of the pituitary gland to secrete oxytocin, which in turn stimulates the myoepithelial cells in the mammary gland to contract and eject the milk (Fig.5.3).

THE NERVE IMPULSE

If the electrical potential between the inside and the outside of an axon is recorded, a potential difference of about 70 millivolts is found, with the inside electrically negative to the outside. This potential difference is known as the resting membrane potential.

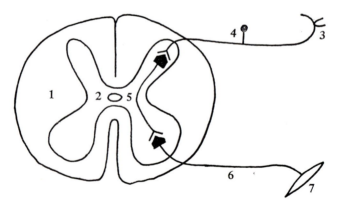

Fig.2.3. Diagram showing the reflex arc. 1) Peripheral white matter containing the nervous tracts. 2) Central gray matter containing the nerve cells. 3) Sense organ. 4) Afferent sensory neuron. 5) Interneuron. 6) Efferent motor neuron. 7) Muscle.

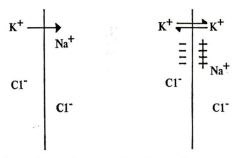

Fig.2.4. Diagram illustrating the origin of a membrane potential (see text).

The membrane potential originates from differences in membrane permeability. Consider a membrane impermeable to Na^+ and Cl^-, but permeable to K^+. The membrane separates two solutions, one is NaCl the other is KCl in equal molar concentrations (Fig.2.4).

Because of the concentration gradient K^+ will move from left to right. Since the other ions cannot cross the membrane, an excess of negative charge will appear on the left side of the membrane. The magnitude of the electrical gradient will depend on the permeability of the membrane to K^+ and of the concentration gradient, and will rise until the electrical gradient pushing K^+ from right to left is equal to the concentration gradient pushing K^+ from left to right.

The actual resting membrane potential of the axon is a result of active transport of Na^+ from inside to outside and active transport of K^+ from outside to inside. These active transport mechanisms create concentration gradients across the membrane and Na^+ will passively move inwards, K^+ passively outwards. Since the membrane is 50 times more permeable to K^+ ions than to Na^+ and practically impermeable to Cl^-, a potential difference will be created leaving the inside of the axon—70 mV negative to the outside (Fig.2.5).

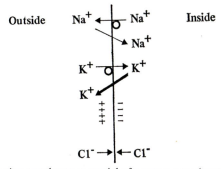

Fig.2.5. The resting membrane potential of a nerve axon (see text).

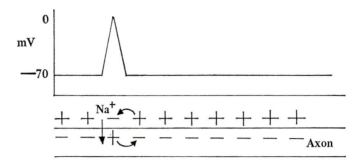

Fig.2.6. The action potential of a nerve axon (see text).

Upon stimulation of the nerve, the membrane momentarily becomes internally positive as a result of increased permeability of the membrane to Na^+. Immediately after depolarization, repolarization begins and Na^+ is actively transported from the inside of the nerve through the membrane to the interstitial fluid surrounding the nerve. The nervous impulse is propagated by setting up local circuits as shown in Fig.2.6. The current flows away from the active region inside the membrane and back again on the outside of the nerve. This current flow depolarizes to a critical level the membrane ahead and creates another active focus. Most mammalian nerves are covered by a myelin sheath interrupted by unmyelinated areas. In such nerves impulses jump from one unmyelinated area to the next and conduction is, therefore, very rapid.

THE AUTONOMIC NERVOUS SYSTEM

The somatic efferent nerves, the motoneurons, have their cell bodies in the spinal cord, and their axons travel without an intervening synapse to the skeletal muscle. All other effector structures in the body are supplied by the autonomic efferent nerves. The autonomic path from the central nervous system to the peripheral structure contains two axons with an intervening synapse. The first axon is termed preganglionic, the second postganglionic. There is no obvious distinction between the somatic and the autonomic afferent nerves.

Another important physiological difference between the autonomic and somatic efferent systems is that in the latter the peripheral synapse is always excitatory. Relaxation of the skeletal muscle is due to lack of activity in the somatic motoneurons, whereas relaxation of smooth and cardiac muscles may be actively brought about by autonomic activity.

The autonomic nervous system is divided into the sympathetic and the parasympathetic system depending on the site of origin of the preganglionic neurons. The sympathetic preganglionic cell bodies are in the intermediate gray matter of the thoracic and lumbar spinal segments. The axons leave the ventral roots in the ordinary way. They then leave the somatic fibres via the rami communicantes and enter the sympathetic chains which run parallel to the vertebral column on each side. Opposite each ventral root there is a swelling known as a ganglion.

There are three main courses open to each preganglionic axon. It may synapse with a postganglionic neuron in its own ganglion and also send branches up and down the chain to synapse other ganglia. It may pass straight through the ganglia into the splanchnic nerves and thereby reach the coeliac and other ganglia lying centrally on the abdominal aorta. Finally the axon may pass to the cells of the adrenal medulla.

The postganglionic fibres innervate the structures outlined in Table 2.1. The function of the sympathetic system is commonly stated to be the preparation of the animal for emergencies. The activation leads to rise in cardiac output and blood pressure, rise in blood glucose concentration, and other changes which prepare the animal for immediate action.

The parasympathetic nerves originate in the nuclei of certain cranial nerves, mainly the vagal nerve, and in the second, third, and fourth sacral nerves. Unlike the sympathetic nerves, they synapse in

Table 2.1 Actions of the autonomic nervous system

Organ	Sympathetic	Parasympathetic
Saliva glands	mucous secretion	serous secretion
Digestive glands	inhibition	secretion
Muscles of hair follicles	contraction	
Muscles of digestive tract	1) inhibition of motility	1) increased motility
	2) contraction of sphincters	2) relaxation of sphincters
Muscles of bronchi	relaxation	contraction
Muscles of bladder	1) contraction of sphincter	1) relaxation of sphincter
	2) relaxation of wall	2) contraction of wall
Heart	increase in rate	decrease in rate
Blood vessels	vasoconstriction	vasodilation

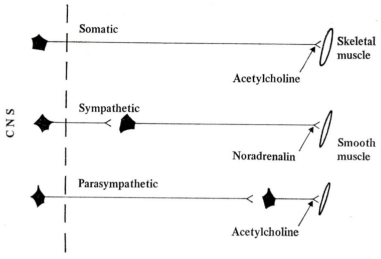

Fig.2.7. Diagram showing the difference between the somatic and the autonomic nervous system (CNS = central nervous system).

the walls of the viscera themselves and not close to the spinal cord. The distribution of parasympathetic nerves is more limited and each preganglionic neuron does not synapse with more than one or two postganglionic ones.

The function of the autonomic nervous system is to help maintain the constancy of the internal environment. The autonomic system regulates the supply of food by controlling the glands and muscles of the gut, the body temperature, the blood glucose concentration, the blood pressure, etc. It is this constancy of the internal environment in face of external changes which enables animals to be independent of surrounding conditions. Usually when an organ is innervated by both sympathetic and parasympathetic fibres the effects of the two are reciprocal. That is, if the sympathetic system excites the organ, the parasympathetic system inhibits it.

The parasympathetic fibres release acetylcholine at the post-ganglionic nerve endings as well as at the synapses between pre-ganglionic and postganglionic neurons. The sympathetic fibres differ from this in that they release noradrenalin at the postganglionic nerve endings. While the acetylcholine is removed momentarily by the enzyme acetylcholine esterase, noradrenalin may circulate in the blood for some time. Therefore, the parasympathetic reaction is short and the sympathetic reaction prolonged (Fig.2.7).

3

Muscular system

Three types of muscle exist in mammals: (1) skeletal or striated muscle moves the skeleton; (2) smooth muscle is found in the walls of hollow organs such as the gastro-intestinal tract, blood vessels, and bladder; (3) cardiac muscle is found only in the heart.

SKELETAL MUSCLE

Muscle cells are specialized for the function of contraction: the contractile mechanism is stimulated by an action potential spreading over the fibre membrane. The action potential is similar to that of nerves. Each skeletal muscle fibre receives the ending of one moto-neuron axon. The junction is a specialized form of synapse known as the neuromuscular junction. Just before the junction, the axon loses its myelin sheath and breaks up into a number of branches. Each branch appears to become partially embedded in the muscle fibre. The nerve endings contain far more mitochondria than the main axon, indicating considerable biochemical activity. The region of the muscle fibre with which the nerve makes contact is known as the end-plate. This contains many nuclei. The muscle membrane on the end-plate contains a series of folds, the junctional folds. There is a cleft, the synaptic cleft, about 500 Å wide which completely separates the nerve from the muscle. Within the nerve endings there are large numbers of synaptic vesicles (Figure 3.1).

When the action potential of the axon reaches the neuromuscular junction it causes the release of a chemical transmitter from the nerve ending. The transmitter is acetylcholine, which increases the permeability of the muscle cell membrane to Na^+, and thus creates an action potential in the same way as in the nerves. The acetylcholine is released from the synaptic vesicles. An enzyme, acetylcholine esterase, destroys the transmitter and terminates the depolarizing action.

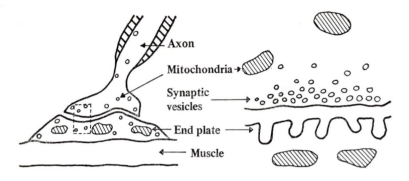

Fig.3.1. The structure of the neuromuscular junction.

Muscular contraction

Each skeletal muscle is made up of a large number of fibres. These
lie parallel to one another and are bound to each other and to the
tendons at each end of the muscle by connective tissue. Each fibre is
bounded by a membrane, the sarcolemma. Within the sarcolemma
there are at least five important types of material, the nuclei, the
sarcoplasm, the sarcoplasmic reticulum, the contractile fibrils, and
the mitochondria. Muscles contain stores of glycogen and the
enzyme systems for its complete oxidation. They also contain the red
pigment myoglobin, which, like haemoglobin, can bind oxygen and
thus acts as an oxygen store.

The striking feature of skeletal muscle fibres when seen under the
high power of a microscope is that they are striated. The striation is
due to differences in the refractive indices of the material in the
fibrils. The main features are a dark A-band with a lighter H-band
in its centre, and a light I-band with a dark Z-line in its centre. The
two main constituents of the fibrils are the proteins actin, the
material of the I-band, and myosin, the material of the A-band
(Fig.3.2).

When the muscle is stimulated bridges are formed between the
actin and the myosin filaments. When these bridges shorten, the
actin and myosin filaments are pulled past each other. The shortened
bridges then break, and new ones are formed which, in turn, shorten
and pull the filaments a little further. When the muscle contracts the
H-band disappears, the I-band decreases, and the A-band remains
unchanged (Fig.3.3).

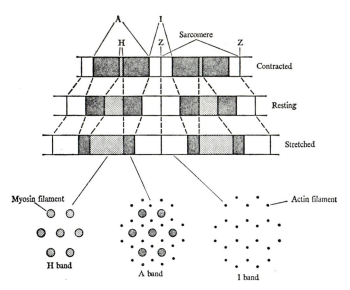

Fig.3.2. The striations of muscle and the charges which they undergo during contraction. The lower figures demonstrate the arrangements of the action and myosin filaments as seen in transverse section with the aid of the electron microscope (from Horrobin, *Medical Physiology and Biochemistry*, by kind permission of the author and Edward Arnold, 1968).

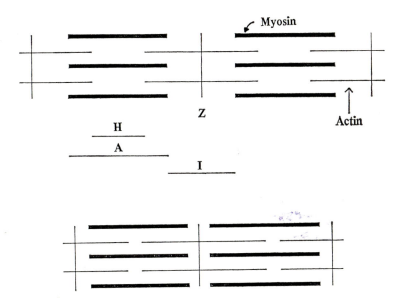

Fig.3.3. Diagram showing relaxed and contracted striated muscle fibres.

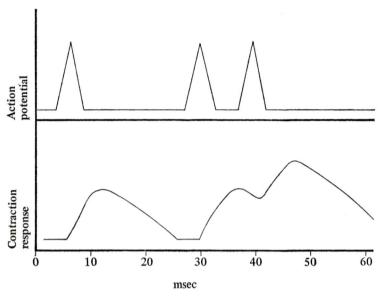

Fig.3.4. The action potential and muscular contraction following single electrical stimulation (see text).

The energy required for muscular contraction is derived from the energy rich compound adenosine triphosphate (ATP). When it splits into adenosine diphosphate (ADP) and phosphoric acid (H_3PO_4) it gives off energy.

The bridges between actin and myosin are formed spontaneously in the absence of ATP, that is when $ATP \rightarrow ADP + H_3PO_4$. In the presence of ATP, when the reaction is reversed, the bridges split and the muscle relaxes. The reaction $ATP \rightarrow ADP + H_3PO_4$ is catalyzed by free myosin. The reverse reaction requires energy, which is obtained from another energy rich compound phosphoryl-creatinine. This compound reacts with ADP to become creatinine.

Phosphorylcreatinine + ADP $\rightleftharpoons$ Creatinine + ATP.

When this process goes from left to right the muscle relaxes, when it goes from right to left the muscle contracts.

Contraction of the whole muscle

If an experiment is performed in which both the action potential of the muscle fibre and the contraction following the stimulation are recorded, the results shown in Figure 3.4 will be obtained. This

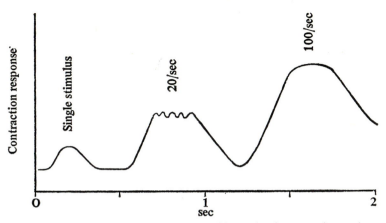

Fig.3.5. The contractile response to stimuli of increasing frequency (see text).

shows what happens when each shock is strong enough to stimulate all the muscle fibres (Fig.3.4).

The action potential is completely over within about 5 msec. The contraction does not begin until 2–3 msec after the beginning of the action potential and lasts from 10–100 msec. It does not reach its peak until after the action potential has finished.

If a second stimulus is given during the contraction period a new contraction will occur and the peak will be higher than the first one.

If the second stimulus is given very shortly after the first there is no time for relaxation between the two contractions since the first one has not even reached its peak. The resulting response is bigger than the response of a single stimulus.

When stimuli follow one another so rapidly that there is no relaxation between them, the resulting response is called a tetanus (Figure 3.5).

SMOOTH MUSCLE

The smooth muscles are physiologically very important. On them depends the function of the gastro-intestinal system, the urinary system, the reproductive system, and the vascular system. The responses of smooth muscle are much more variable than those of skeletal muscle and less well understood.

The normal membrane potential is in the region of -60 mV, but may vary in size. The action potentials also vary in size, and are accompanied by increases in tension, proportional to the extent of the potential change.

Smooth muscle cells either respond to noradrenaline released by the sympathetic nerves or to acetylcholine released by the parasympathetic nerves. If a specific smooth muscle cell is caused to contract by sympathetic stimulation, either it will not respond at all to parasympathetic stimulation or it will relax.

There are two types of smooth muscle: both contain actin and myosin and it seems likely that the basic mechanism of contraction of both of these is the same as in skeletal muscle. The arrangement of the proteins, however, is much less regular than in skeletal muscle. The two types are known as visceral and multi-unit muscle.

Visceral muscle is found in the wall of the gastro-intestinal tract. The resting membrane potential is normally in the region of -50 mV, but there are repeated miniature depolarizations, some of which are sufficient to initiate an action potential. Stretching the muscle fibre tends to depolarize it, to increase the frequency of action potentials and to increase the tension developed by the fibre. In visceral smooth muscle acetylcholine tends to depolarize the membrane further, resulting in a higher frequency of action potentials and thus a greater development of tension. The action of adrenalin is more complex. It inhibits contraction of some visceral smooth muscle and stimulates the contraction of others. The structure of adrenalin is such that it occupies two different types of receptors on smooth muscle. The filling of the α receptors produces one type of response, usually excitation, while the occupation of β receptors produces another type, usually inhibition. Whether adrenalin produces excitation or inhibition depends on the balance of the two types of receptors on the particular tissue in question.

Multi-unit smooth muscle is found in places where finely graded contractions are essential, such as in the iris of the eye and the walls of the blood vessels. Its fibres have a relatively stable membrane potential and normally require nervous stimulation if they are to contract. Acetylcholin is excitatory while adrenalin can have either α or β effects, depending on which muscle it acts.

The smooth muscle differs from skeletal muscle in the fact that there is no rapid mechanism for the destruction of transmitters at the neuromuscular junction. Their contractions therefore tend to be prolonged.

4

Sense organs

Information about the internal and external environment is relayed to the central nervous system from the various sense organs. Within these organs are receptor cells which convert various forms of energy in the environment into action potentials in the sensory nerves. The forms of energy converted by the receptors include, for example, mechanical (pressure or touch), thermal (heat or cold), electromagnetic (light), and chemical energy (odour, taste, oxygen and carbon dioxide content of the blood). The receptors in each of these sense organs are adapted to respond to one particular form of energy at a much lower threshold than other receptors respond to this form of energy.

GENERAL SENSATION

General sensory information is relayed from exterior and interior receptors. The exterior receptors react to changes in the external environment. They are located in the skin and in the special senses. The sensation of pain originates in the free nerve endings in the epidermis and subcutis, whereas the sensation of touch is relayed from the Meissner's corpuscles of the connective tissue deep in the epidermis, and from the Merkel's discs of the lips and muzzle. Deeper in the subcutaneous tissue are found the Pacinian corpuscles which are connected with the sensation of deep pressure. Differences in surrounding temperature may be sensed by the Ruffini corpuscles (heat) and the Krause end bulbs (cold). These organs are found in the connective tissue.

The interior receptors (proprioceptors) react to changes in the internal environment. Important for the co-ordination of body movements are the proprioceptors in muscle. The receptors are located in the muscles and joints and indicate to the animal the relative position of various parts of the body without the use of the eyes. Sensation of pain due to lack of blood supply, distension or contraction is relayed by receptors in the viscera.

TASTE

The sensation of taste is related to the taste buds, which are barrel-shaped cell groups consisting of fusiform gustatory cells intermingled with supporting cells. Hair-like processes of the gustatory cells project through a pore at the superficial portion of the taste-bud. The nerve fibres terminate around the gustatory cells (Fig.4.1).

The taste-buds are found in large numbers in the mucous membrane of the tongue and the pharynx.

The four specific taste modalities include sweet, salt, bitter, and sour. All taste sensation involves mixtures of these basic tastes or combinations of tastes and smell.

SMELL

Olfactory nerve cells are scattered among columnar supporting cells throughout the mucous membrane in the dorsal and caudal part of the nasal cavity. The nucleus of each olfactory cell is located near the basement membrane of the mucous membrane. A peripheral process extends between supporting cells to the surface, where it bears a tuft of several fine hair-like projections which are assumed to be the actual receptors for the sense of smell. Since these processes are normally covered by moist mucus, the material to be smelled must probably go into solution before it can reach the sensory cells.

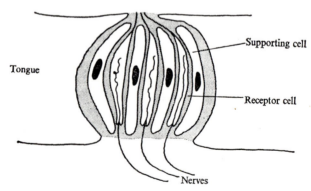

Fig.4.1. The structure of a taste bud (from Horrobin, *Medical Physiology and Biochemistry*, by kind permission of the author and Edward Arnold, 1968).

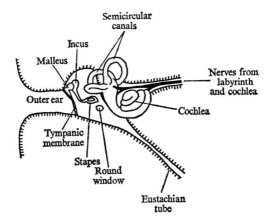

Fig.4.2. Outline of the structure of the ear (from Horrobin, *Medical Physiology and Biochemistry*, by kind permission of the author and Edward Arnold, 1968).

FUNCTIONS OF THE EAR

Receptors for hearing and equilibrium are housed in the ear. The external ear, the middle ear and the cochlea of the inner ear are concerned with hearing. The semicircular canals, the utricle, and the saccule of the inner ear are concerned with equilibrium.

The external ear extends from the exterior to the tympanic membrane. The middle ear is an air-filled cavity in the temporal bone which communicates with the pharynx via the Eustachian tube. It is separated from the external ear by the tympanic membrane and from the inner ear by the membranes which close the oval and the round window. The three auditory ossicles (malleus, incus, and stapes) provide the mechanical linkage from the tympanic membrane to the membrane closing the oval window. Two small skeletal muscles are also located in the middle ear. Their function is to decrease the vibrations of the membranes. The inner ear is made up of two parts, one within the other. The bony labyrinth is a series of canals in the petrous bone. Inside these canals, surrounded by a fluid called perilymph, is the membranous labyrinth. The membranous labyrinth is more or less a duplicate of the shape of the bony canals. It is filled with a fluid called endolymph, and there is no communication between the spaces filled with endolymph and those filled with perilymph.

The cochlear portion of the labyrinth is a coiled tube divided into three chambers. The upper and lower chambers or scalae contain

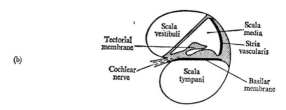

Fig.4.3. Transverse section of the cochlea (from Horrobin, *Medical Physiology and Biochemistry*, by kind permission of the author and Edward Arnold, 1968).

perilymph and communicate with each other at the apex of the cochlea. The upper chamber ends in the oval window, the lower in the round window. The middle cochlear chamber is continuous with the membranous labyrinth and does not communicate with the two other chambers. It contains endolymph (Fig.4.3).

Located on the membrane which separates the middle and lower chambers, and extending into the middle chamber, is the organ of Corti. This organ extends from the apex to the base of the cochlea, and consequently has a spiral shape. The organ of Corti contains the auditory receptors which are hair cells. They increase in length from the base of the cochlea to the apex. From the auditory receptor cells afferent nerves carry auditory impulses to the brain (Fig.4.4)

When sound waves strike the tympanic membrane they are transferred mechanically by the ossicles to the membrane of the oval window. Pressure on this membrane is transmitted throughout all the perilymph and endolymph. Since the fluid is incompressible, any movement of the oval membrane must be compensated by an opposite movement of the round membrane. The hair cells in the organ

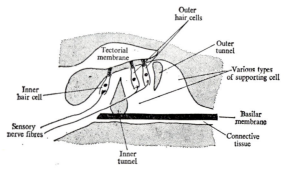

Fig.4.4. The structure of the organ of Corti (from Horrobin, *Medical Physiology and Biochemistry*, by kind permission of the author and Edward Arnold, 1968).

of Corti vibrate in resonance with the frequency of the sound waves entering the ear. Impulses from the vibrating portion of the cochlea are transmitted by the acoustic nerve to reach a spot on the cerebral cortex that corresponds with the frequency and consequently with the frequency of the original sound wave striking the ear.

On each side of the head, the semicircular canals are perpendicular to each other so that they are orientated in the three planes of space. Inside the bony canals, the membranous canals are suspended in the perilymph. A receptor structure is located in the extended end or ampulla of each of the membranous canals. The receptors consist of hair cells from which afferent fibres go to the brain. Also in other parts of the membranous labyrinth, the utricle and the saccule, equilibrium receptors are found. The receptor cells are surmounted by a membrane in which are embedded crystals of calcium carbonate, the otoliths.

The vestibular receptors are stimulated by the movement of the endolymph and the otoliths in response to rotational and linear acceleration of the body.

VISION

The eye consists of two segments of a sphere, a larger segment and a smaller called the cornea, or transparent anterior part of the eye. The outer layer of the large segment is known as the sclera. The next layer is the vascular tunic and includes the choroid, ciliary body, and iris. The deepest layer is the nervous tunic known as the retina. It is the origin of the optic nerve and contains the rods and cones which are receptive to light. The impulses received on the retina are transmitted by way of the optic nerve to the brain, where they are interpreted as visual images (Fig.4.5).

The interior of the eye is filled with a gelatinous material, the vitreous humour. In front of this the lens is located, surrounded by the ciliary body. Focusing the lens—accommodation—is accomplished by means of contraction or relaxation of the ciliary muscle. The iris forms a curtain to control the amount of light entering the eye. The pupil of the eye is the opening in the centre of the iris.

The light rays from an object are focused on the retina to produce an inverted image. The retina contains two types of receptors for light, cones which differentiate colours, and rods which allow vision under low illumination.

Rhodopsin is the pigment involved in the photochemical change

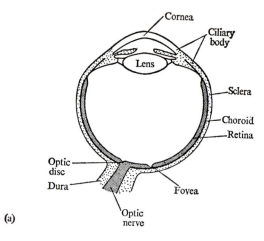

(a)

that translates light waves into nerve impulses in the rods. The compound is synthesized from retinene and a protein molecule in the relative absence of light. Retinene in turn is reduced to vitamin A by the enzyme alcohol dehydrogenase.

$$\underset{\substack{\text{(purple)}}}{\text{Rhodopsin}} \underset{\text{dark}}{\overset{\text{light}}{\rightleftharpoons}} \underset{\text{(yellow)}}{\text{Retinene}} + \text{protein} \underset{\text{dark}}{\overset{\substack{\text{alcohol dehydrogenase} \\ \text{light}}}{\rightleftharpoons}} \text{Vitamin A} + \text{protein}$$

The cones are able to distinguish between light rays of different wavelengths. There are said to be three different types of cones, reacting to red, green, and blue. Other colours are perceived because of mixtures of the combined responses of these three.

5

Endocrine system

An endocrine gland produces a chemical substance (hormone) which is carried by the blood to a target organ at some distance from the gland. The endocrine system is related to the nervous system in that both serve the same purpose: to act as the communication system between different organs, and thus regulate their physiological and biochemical functions. The sympathetic nerves, for example, produce noradrenalin, a substance similar to that produced by the adrenal medulla. It is difficult to classify one substance as a hormone and not the other, because they have so many similarities, and yet one fits the definition and the other does not.

The proof of the presence of a hormone consists of experimental removal of the gland believed to produce the hormone in question. If this operation is always followed by the same symptoms, and if these symptoms can be relieved by appropriate extracts of the gland, a hormone is regarded as proven as a product of the specific gland.

Endocrine glands are usually slower and more sustained in their action than the nervous system. Some reflexes involve nerves on the afferent side and hormones on the efferent side of the reflex arc (ovulation following coitus in rabbits, the suckling stimulus and milk let down in cows).

Some hormones affect all body tissues, whereas others act on one organ or gland in particular, the target organ. Hormone production is often the result of an interaction between different endocrine organs, interaction between a trophic hormone and its target organ. The trophic hormones are generally stimulating in nature, causing the target organ to release increased amounts of its own hormone. As well as acting on the body cells in general, this target gland hormone also acts at the site of trophic hormone production to inhibit further production of the trophin. This mechanism is known as a negative feed-back mechanism.

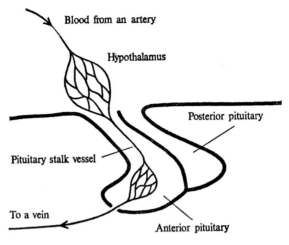

Fig.5.1. The pituitary gland and its blood supply (Horrobin).

The action of the hormones on the cellular level is not very well understood. It seems, however, that hormones participate in the intracellular enzymatic processes as enzyme activators. They are further known to alter the properties of the cell membrane, and thus the exchange of compounds between the intracellular fluids.

THE PITUITARY GLAND

The pituitary gland is located at the base of the brain in the sella turcica, a depression in the floor of the cranial cavity. The gland consists of an anterior lobe, an intermediate lobe, and a posterior lobe. The posterior lobe originates from the embryonic brain and is in the adult still connected to the brain by means of the pituitary stalk. Many nerves go from the hypothalamus down to the posterior pituitary.

The blood supply of the pituitary gland originates in the internal carotid artery. Some branches go directly to the gland, whereas others go to a capillary system in the hypothalamus. From these capillaries the blood passes through a few venules to the capillary system of the pituitary gland. Via this vascular system, known as the hypothalamic–pituitary portal system, the neurohormones or releasing factors are carried from the hypothalamus to the pituitary gland. The releasing factors regulate the production of the various pituitary hormones (Fig.5.1)

The nerves that enter the anterior pituitary gland probably control vessel size rather than cause glandular secretion directly.

Anterior lobe hormones

Somatotrophin or growth hormone (STH) stimulates growth of all body tissues, being particularly effective with respect to bone and muscle tissue. Excess of STH in the immature animal results in overall excess growth, including longer limbs, and produces a giant individual. In the mature animal the extremities enlarge in diameter but not in length. Deficiency of STH is seen in hypophysectomized (pituitary gland removed) young animals. These animals become dwarfs. The biochemical mechanism of STH is not clear. There seems to be a direct effect on the synthesis of protein, on the breakdown of triglycerides, and on utilization of free fatty acids in preference to glucose.

The secretion of STH is controlled by a releasing factor in response to the blood glucose level. Low blood glucose concentration stimulates the hypothalamus to produce the releasing factor which travels down the pituitary stalk blood vessels and stimulates the pituitary gland to secrete the somatotrophin. High blood glucose concentrations depress the secretion of the hormone.

Prolactin (LTH) is important for the initiation and maintenance of milk secretion. The secretion of the hormone is stimulated by the high levels of oestrogen in the blood, whereas the action of the hormone on the mammary gland is inhibited by progesterone. These two hormones are produced by the foetal membranes in the last part of pregnancy. After parturition the inhibiting action of progesterone disappears, and milk secretion commences. The release of LTH is also reflexly stimulated by suckling.

Thyrotrophin or thyroid stimulating hormone (TSH) has its primary action on the thyroid gland. Thyroid epithelial cells undergo hypertrophy and hyperplasia, and the production and release of thyroid hormone increases under the influence of TSH. The release of TSH is regulated by a negative feed-back mechanism. If the thyroid gland is removed, the amount of thyroid hormone in the blood falls and the output of TSH increases. When, on the other hand large doses of thyroid hormone are administered to an animal, the TSH output will decrease.

The adrenocorticotrophic hormone (ACTH) stimulates the adrenal cortex, but not the adrenal medulla. In the cortex the ACTH

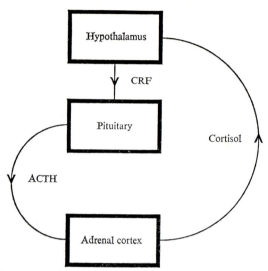

Fig.5.2. The control of ACTH and cortisol levels (Horrobin).

stimulates the cells producing glucocorticoids, but not cells producing mineralocorticoids. The release of ACTH is controlled by the hypothalamus, from where an ACTH releasing factor is secreted and brought by way of the hypothalamic-pituitary system to the ACTH producing cells in the anterior lobe of the pituitary gland. The production of the ACTH releasing factor is regulated by a negative feed-back mechanism involving the concentration of glucocorticoid in the blood (Fig.5.2).

Follicle stimulating hormone (FSH) causes follicles in the ovary to develop and enlarge. In the presence of luteinizing hormone (LH) the follicles will mature and oestrogen will be produced. As the level of circulating oestrogen increases, production of FSH is inhibited by a negative feed-back mechanism. As FSH production decreases, LH production increases with the result that the follicle matures and ovulates.

LH is correlated with maturation of the ovum, ovulation and formation of the corpus luteum. The corpus luteum produces the hormone progesterone, which not only inhibits production of LH but also prevents follicle growth and ovulation, thus preventing oestrus during the life of the corpus luteum. In the male animal LH acts on the hormone producing cells in the testes, the interstitial cells. The hormone is therefore known as the interstitial cell stimula-

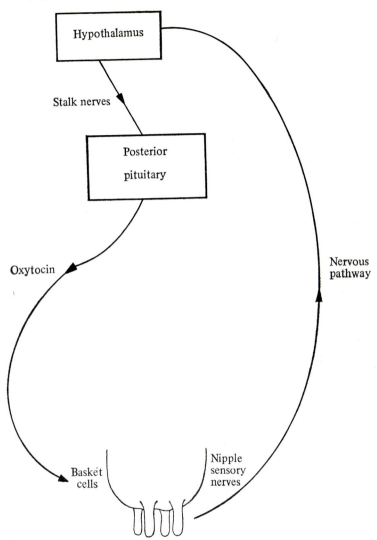

Fig.5.3. The control of milk ejection. The myoepithelial cells are sometimes known as basket cells.

ting hormone (ICSH) in males. The interstitial cells produce the male hormone testosterone.

Intermediate lobe hormones

The intermediate lobe of the pituitary gland produces the melanocyte stimulating hormone (MSH). This hormone is associated with the control of pigment cells in lower forms of animals. The hormone causes darkening of the skin in these animals.

Posterior lobe hormones

The actual source of posterior lobe hormones are the nerve cells of the hypothalamus. From here the hormones are carried along the nerve axons that pass from the hypothalamus to the posterior lobe, where they are stored until released. The hormones are the antidiuretic hormone and oxytocin.

The antidiuretic hormone (ADH) has an important function in control of water loss from the kidney by facilitating reabsorption of water from the distal portion of the nephron. Lack of ADH causes a disease called diabetes insipidus which is characterized by excess loss of fluid via the kidneys. The release of the hormone is controlled by the osmotic pressure of the blood reaching the osmoreceptors in the hypothalamus. An increased osmotic pressure inhibits the ADH release, whereas a decreased osmotic pressure in the blood has the opposite effect.

Oxytocin acts in the female by stimulating the motility of the uterus and causes contraction of the myoepithelial cells in the mammary gland. The action on the uterus is of importance for the transport of spermatozoa to the site of fertilization, and of importance for the act of parturition. The effect of oxytocin on the myometrium is under the influence of other hormones. The oestrogens increase the action of oxytocin, and progesterone inhibits it. Suckling causes reflex release of oxytocin, which causes the myoepithelial cells surrounding the alveoli of the mammary gland to contract. This process, known as 'milk let down' forces milk out of the alveoli into the ducts of the mammary gland. Washing the teats before milking the cow causes the same reflex (Fig.5.3).

In the male animal oxytocin stimulates motility of the epididymis and the vas deferens, and thus aids the transport of semen during ejaculation.

THE THYROID GLAND

The thyroid gland maintains in the tissues a level of metabolism which is optimal for their function. Thyroid hormone stimulates the O_2 consumption of most cells in the body, helps to regulate lipid and carbohydrate metabolism, and is necessary for normal growth and

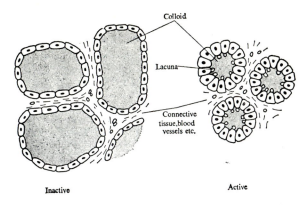

Fig.5.4. Active and inactive thyroid tissue (Horrobin).

maturation. Thyroid function is controlled by the thyroid stimulating hormone (TSH) of the anterior pituitary, and the secretion of this trophic hormone is in turn regulated by a direct inhibitory feedback of high circulating thyroid hormone levels.

The thyroid gland consists of two lobes located near the thyroid cartilage of the larynx. An isthmus may or may not connect the two lobes varying with the species. A connective tissue capsule covers the gland and sends into it septa which gives support and conducts vessels to the epithelial cells. The gland is well vascularized and has one of the highest rates of blood flow per gram of tissue of any organ in the body. The thyroid is made up of multiple follicles. Each follicle is surrounded by a single layer of cells and filled with a proteinaceous material called colloid. When the gland is inactive the colloid is abundant, the follicles are large and the cells lining them are flat. When the gland is active the follicles are small and the cells are columnar. The individual thyroid cells rest on a basement membrane which separates them from the adjacent capillaries (Fig.5.4).

The principal hormone secreted by the thyroid gland is thyroxin, an iodine-containing amino acid. Small amounts of triiodothyronine and other compounds are also liberated. Thyroxin is synthesized in the colloid by iodination and condensation of tyrosine molecules that are bound in peptide linkage to thyroglobulin (Fig.5.5). The thyroxin remains in this bound form until it is secreted. During secretion, the peptide bonds are hydrolyzed and free thyroxin enters the thyroid cells, crosses them, and is discharged into the capillaries.

The thyroid hormone requires iodine as an essential part of the

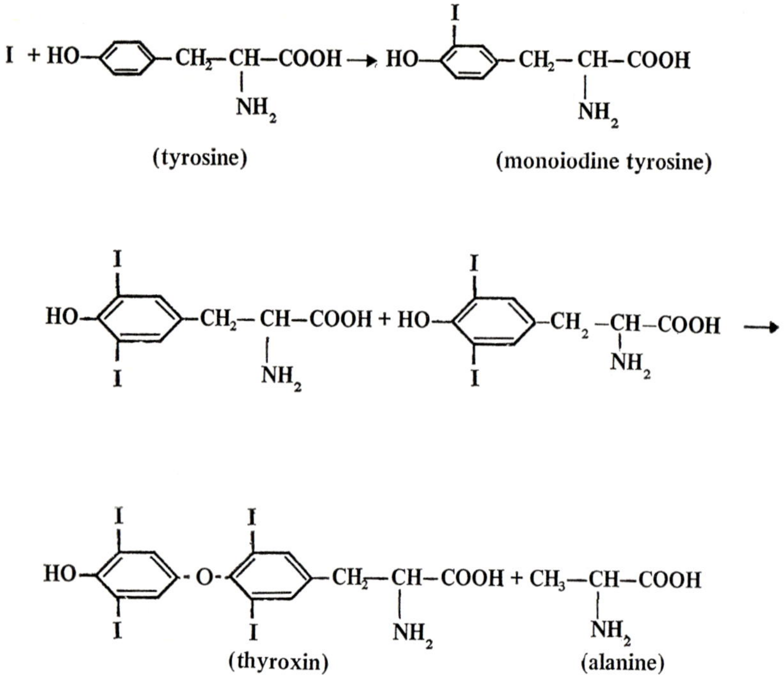

Fig.5.5. Outline of thyroxin synthesis.

molecule. The thyroid gland has a remarkable ability to absorb iodine from the blood. The intracellular concentration of iodine is 20 to 40 times that of the circulating blood. The mechanism of this iodine pump is not known, but it can be inhibited by thiocyanates and other compounds.

When thyroxin is released into the blood it is bound to an alpha-globulin fraction known as the thyroxin binding globulin (TBG). The plasma protein bound iodine (PBI) amounts to 4–7 μg per 100 ml. In cases of hypo-function of the thyroid gland it is decreased to 3–4 μg per cent, and in hyper-function it increases to 15–20 μg per cent.

The thyroid hormone influences enzymatic processes throughout the body, mainly transphosphorylations. In this way the hormone stimulates absorption of glucose from the intestine and mobilization of glycogen from the liver. The site of action of the thyroid hormone is the mitochondria, which contain the enzymes of the aerobic pathways of carbohydrate and lipid metabolism. There may also be

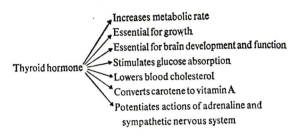

Thyroid hormone
- Increases metabolic rate
- Essential for growth
- Essential for brain development and function
- Stimulates glucose absorption
- Lowers blood cholesterol
- Converts carotene to vitamin A
- Potentiates actions of adrenaline and sympathetic nervous system

Fig.5.6. The main actions of thyroid hormone (Horrobin).

other sites of action as well. The main effects are summarized in Figure 5.6.

Lack of thyroid hormone in the young animal causes a dwarfing condition called cretinism. In the adult animal hypothyroidism results in lower metabolic rate, decreased heart action, lower blood pressure, and decreased urine secretion. The decreased metabolism also affects the nervous system and the muscles, resulting in general depression. The interstitial fluid volume increases owing to retention of Na^+ and Cl^-. Hypothyroidism also leads to disfunction of the gonads, known as summer sterility in cows, and to reduction in milk production.

A deficiency of iodine in the diet over an extended period of time will cause enlargement of the thyroid gland, a condition known as goitre. Owing to low concentration of iodine in the blood, the production of thyroxin will be low. In response to this the production of TSH from the pituitary gland increases, leading to hypertrophy of the thyroid gland and better utilization of the iodine. If the iodine deficiency occurs during pregnancy the foetus may become abnormal (hairless and blind calves).

In addition to iodine deficiency, certain compounds may produce goitre, either by blocking the uptake of iodine by the thyroid gland or by blocking the formation of the hormone.

Hyperthyroidism, or excess thyroid activity, is associated with increased metabolic rate, increased heart rate, loss of weight with a normal or increased appetite, irritability, and nervousness.

THE PARATHYROID GLAND

The hormone secreted by the parathyroid glands raises the plasma calcium level, mobilizes calcium from bone, and increases urinary phosphate excretion. The rate of secretion of the parathyroid hormone varies inversely with the plasma calcium level.

The parathyroid glands are small nodules located within or near the thyroid gland. Commonly there are two parathyroid glands on each side, but the exact number and location varies with the species.

The parathyroid hormone is essential for life. Removal of the gland results in a low ionic calcium concentration in the blood and urine, with a concurrent increase in phosphorus in the blood and reduced phosphorus in the urine. Blood calcium falls from the normal 9–11 mg per 100 ml to as low as 5 mg per 100 ml. Low ionic calcium blood level affects the neuromuscular system, leading, in increasing severity, from twitchings to tremors and spasms of the muscles (tetany) to convulsions and finally to death.

An excess of the parathyroid hormone causes an increased mobilization of calcium from the skeleton. Calcium may reach as high a level as 20 mg per 100 ml in the blood, whereas the phosphorus concentration falls. There is also an increased calcium and phosphorus excretion in the urine. Continued withdrawal of calcium from the skeleton causes it to become softened and weak and subject to deformities.

Calcium in the blood is found partly bound to protein and partly as free ionized calcium. The ionized calcium is necessary for blood coagulation, normal cardiac and skeletal muscle contraction, and normal nerve function. Plasma proteins are more ionized when the pH is high, providing more protein anions to bind with calcium. Thus tetany is more likely when blood is alkaline. The calcium in bone is partly in the form of a readily exchangeable reservoir, and partly as a larger pool of stable calcium that is only slowly exchangeable. The plasma calcium is in equilibrium with the readily exchangeable bone calcium.

The absorption of calcium from the intestinal tract takes place by an active mechanism and is dependent on vitamin D. Injection of large doses of this vitamin causes a rise in blood calcium level. Parathyroid hormone may have a minor role in calcium absorption.

The parathyroid hormone has two main functions, mobilization of calcium from the skeleton and increased phosphate excretion in the urine (Fig.5.7). The way the hormone acts on bone is not known in detail. It seems to stimulate the formation of certain cells, osteoclasts, which are known to break down bone tissue. The effect on the kidneys is not due to any change in the amount of phosphate filtered in the glomeruli, and it is not known whether it is due to a decrease

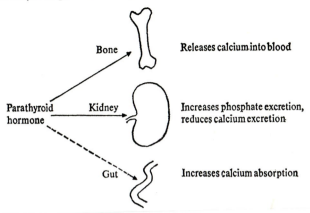

Fig.5.7. The actions of parathyroid hormone (Horrobin).

in tubular reabsorption or an increase in tubular secretion of phosphate.

Normal control of secretion of the parathyroid hormone depends largely on the level of ionized calcium in the blood and is independent of the pituitary gland (Fig.5.8). When the calcium level is high, secretion is inhibited, and calcium is deposited in the bones. When it is low, secretion is increased, and calcium is mobilized from the bones.

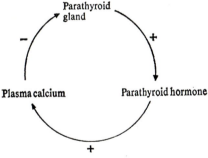

Fig.5.8. The control of the parathyroid hormone excretion (Horrobin).

Calcitonin

The hormone calcitonin is secreted from the thyroid gland and its output is controlled by the calcium concentration of the blood. Calcitonin acts on the skeleton, where it inhibits the mobilization of calcium and phosphorus, i.e. it thus lowers plasma calcium levels. The hormone has no direct effect on absorption or excretion of calcium and phosphorus.

ADRENAL GLAND HORMONES

There are two endocrine organs in the adrenal gland, one surrounding the other in most species. The inner adrenal medulla secretes adrenalin and noradrenalin. The outer adrenal cortex secretes steroid hormones.

The adrenal medulla is in effect a sympathetic ganglion in which the postganglionic neurons have lost their axons and become secretory cells. The cells secrete when stimulated by the preganglionic fibres that reach the gland via the splanchnic nerves. Adrenal medullary hormones are not essential for life, but they prepare the individual to deal with emergencies.

The adrenal cortex secretes glucocorticoids, steroids with widespread effects on the metabolism of carbohydrates and proteins, mineralocorticoids which are essential to the maintenance of both sodium balance and extracellular fluid volume, and sex hormones which exert minor effects on reproductive functions. Unless mineralocorticoid and glucocorticoid replacement therapy is administered post-operatively, removal of the adrenal glands is followed by collapse and death.

Adrenal medulla

Noradrenalin and adrenalin are both secreted by the adrenal medulla. Noradrenalin is formed by hydroxylation and decarboxylation of the amino acid phenylalanine, and adrenaline by methylation of noradrenalin. In the resting animal the secretion of noradrenalin and adrenalin is very low and subsequently the blood concentration is low. If the animal is excited or placed under physical stress the secretion from the adrenal medulla increases. The hormones are quickly moved from the blood to the tissues where they are inactivated by other methylation reactions. Excretion takes place via the kidneys and the liver.

The adrenal medulla hormones have a wide range of biological effects. These may be divided into effects on the heart and circulatory system, effects on smooth muscles in other organs, and effects on metabolism.

Adrenalin increases the heart rate and the force with which the heart contracts, the minute volume, and coronary blood flow. Noradrenalin does not show this effect. Injection of noradrenalin causes contraction of the smooth muscles of the arterioles, thus increasing the peripheral resistance and the systolic blood pressure. As a reflex response to the rise in pressure the heart slows down.

Table 5.1 Effect of intravenous injection of adrenalin and noradrenalin. (+) indicates increased action, (0) no action, and (−) decreased action

Effect on:	*Adrenalin*	*Noradrenalin*
Heart rate	+	−
Minute volume	+++	O
Systolic blood pressure	+++	+++
Peripheral resistance	0	++
Oxygen consumption	++	0
Blood glucose concentration	+++	0
Blood lactic acid conc.	+++	0
Gastro-intestinal motility	− − −	− − −
Bronchial muscles	− − −	0

Adrenalin and noradrenalin inhibit the motility of the gastro-intestinal tract except for the sphincter pylori which contracts. Adrenalin also causes relaxation of the bronchial muscles.

Injection of adrenalin causes a rise in the blood glucose and lactic acid concentrations due to increased glycogenolysis in the liver and decreased glucose uptake by peripheral tissues. This effect on the carbohydrate metabolism is accompanied by an increase in the oxygen consumption and the heat production.

Stimulation of a certain area of the brain increases the release of adrenalin and noradrenalin. This stimulation is initiated by the chemoreceptors in response to a fall in the blood glucose concentration. The hormones are also secreted in response to cooling of the skin, painful conditions, and physical or mental stress. Whatever the stimuli, they seem to be coordinated by the same centre in the brain.

Generally speaking the adrenal medulla hormones prepare the animal for quick responses to changes in the environment. The action of the hormones brings the animal to a state of alertness, glucose is mobilized, the oxygen consumption increases, the bronchi expand, the blood can carry more oxygen due to splenic contraction, the action of the heart is increased, and the blood flow through the muscles is increased. Because of these properties the adrenal medulla hormones are often referred to as 'fight or flight hormones'.

Adrenal cortex

The hormones of the adrenal cortex are derivatives of cholesterol. Chemically they are steroids, that is, they are built around the steroid nucleus.

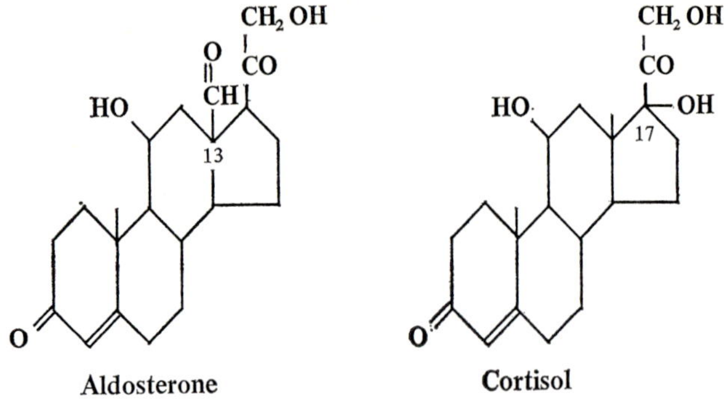

Fig.5.9. The chemical configuration of aldosterone and cortisol. Both hormones are built around the steroid nucleus.

The cortical hormones can be divided into three groups, the mineralocorticoids which are primarily concerned with salt and water metabolism, the glucocorticoids which deal with carbohydrate, fat, and protein metabolism, and the androgens which are male sex hormones.

Mineralocorticoids

The most important mineralocorticoid is aldosterone. The molecule has an aldehyde group at the position C-13. Aldosterone regulates sodium retention and potassium excretion in the kidneys and the salivary glands, and increases sodium absorption in the gastro-intestinal tract.

If aldosterone is given to an animal daily for some time the concentration of sodium in the extracellular fluid space will increase and the concentration of potassium will decrease. The result will be isotonic expansion of the extracellular fluid space.

Following adrenalectomy the animal fails to reabsorb sodium, and therefore becomes depleted of sodium. The sodium concentration of the extracellular fluid space falls and the potassium concentration increases, resulting in loss of water from the extracellular fluid space.

The secretion of aldosterone is only partially dependent on ACTH, and removal of the pituitary gland changes the hormone secretion little. The secretion is also partly regulated by the level of sodium and potassium in the blood. Low sodium and high potassium increases aldosterone output. The most important controlling

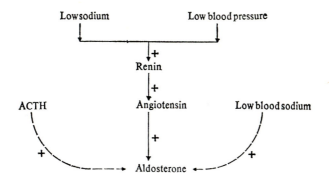

Fig.5.10. The ways in which aldosterone output may be controlled (Horrobin).

mechanism may be an enzyme, renin, which is secreted by the kidney in response to low body sodium levels and a low blood pressure. Renin acts on a plasma protein to form angiotensin and angiotensin stimulates the adrenal cortex to secrete aldosterone (Fig.5.10).

Glucocorticoids

The major glucocorticoid hormone is cortisol (hydrocortisone). The molecule has a hydroxyl group at C-17. Cortisol affects glucose metabolism. Given to a normal animal it increases the blood glucose concentration and the amount of glycogen in the liver. The reason for this is decreased glucose break-down as well as increased gluconeogenesis (synthesis of glucose from protein). If the adrenal glands

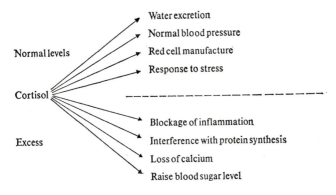

Fig.5.11. The main actions of cortisol (Horrobin).

are removed, liver glycogen and blood glucose fall because of increased glucose metabolism and decreased gluconeogenesis. Cortisol has several other complex actions which are summarized in Figure 5.11.

The secretion of glucocorticoids is regulated by ACTH by means of a feed-back mechanism (Fig. 5.12). An increase in the blood concentration of the hormone inhibits the release of ACTH, and a fall in the hormone concentration in the blood stimulates ACTH production.

Adrenal androgens

Androgens are the hormones that exert masculinizing effects, and they promote protein anabolism and growth. Testosterone from the testes is the most active androgen, and the adrenal androgens have less than one fifth of its activity. Secretion of the adrenal androgens is controlled by ACTH and not by gonadotrophins. The amounts of adrenal androgens secreted are almost as great in castrated males and females as in normal males, but they exert no significant masculiniz-ing effect when secreted in normal amounts. When excess androgen secretion occurs in genetically female foetuses, the development of male type external genitalia is stimulated and various degrees of pseudohermaphroditism result. This condition is commonly seen in pigs.

THE PANCREAS

The islets of Langerhans in the pancreas secrete the polypeptide hormone glucagon and the protein hormone insulin, both of which have important functions in the regulation of intermediary metab-olism. Glucagon elevates blood glucose by stimulating hepatic glycogenolysis, and insulin lowers the blood glucose by facilitating the entry of glucose into muscle and other tissues.

The islets of Langerhans are ovoid collections of cells scattered throughout the pancreas. They make up 1–2 per cent of the weight of the gland. Two hormone producing types of cells are found in the islets, alpha-cells that produce glucagon, and beta-cells that produce insulin. The function of the third type of cells, gamma-cells, is unknown.

Insulin

Removal of the pancreas leads to diabetes mellitus, a disease caused by lack of insulin. The most obvious effect of insulin shortage is a sharp rise in the concentration of blood glucose to about 150–500 mg per 100 ml. The normal value for simple stomach animals is about 100 mg per 100 ml and for ruminants about 60 mg per cent. When the blood glucose concentration passes the renal threshold, which is 160–180 mg per cent, glucose is excreted in the urine. Without insulin there is a much reduced ability to metabolize glucose to carbon dioxide and water, and to synthesize fat from glucose. Glycogen stores in the liver and muscles are low, and resynthesis is slow in the absence of insulin. Since the large amount of glucose in the blood cannot be effectively used by the tissues, both fat and protein serve as energy sources in the diabetic animal, resulting in wasting away of body tissues. The blood contains greater amounts of fat and products of incomplete metabolism of fat and protein.

In the pancreatectomized animal nearly all of the diabetic tendency can be corrected by the administration of insulin, and the animal kept alive in relatively good health if the diet is suitable.

There are three routes of glucose loss in the body: (1) glucose may pass into the cells whose membranes are freely permeable to it. Once inside the cell it may be stored as glycogen or metabolized. This takes place in the liver; (2) glucose may also pass into the cells which are partially impermeable to glucose and be stored or metabolized. The rate limiting step in the glucose metabolism in these cells appears to be the passage across the cell membrane. Until the glucose concentration in the extracellular fluid reaches a certain level, the tissue threshold, no glucose will enter the cell at all. The glucose tissue threshold is not a fixed and immutable property. It can be lowered by several factors such as insulin, oxygen lack, and muscular work. Other factors may increase the tissue threshold. They include growth hormone, adrenalin, glucocorticoids, and non-esterified fatty acids (NEFA); (3) finally, glucose may escape into the urine. With normal kidneys and normal blood glucose concentrations, all the glucose filtered in the glomerulus is reabsorbed and none is excreted from the body. However, if the blood glucose becomes abnormally high, or if the kidney is damaged, the urine may represent a serious route of sugar loss (Fig.5.13).

The biochemical action of insulin is not completely known. The hormone lowers the blood glucose concentration by lowering the tissue threshold for glucose, and hence increasing the rate of glucose uptake by peripheral tissues. Insulin also acts by decreasing the output of glucose from the liver by stimulating glycogen synthesis.

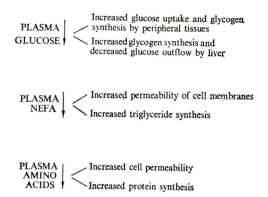

Fig.5.12. Summary of the actions of insulin (from Horrobin, *Medical Physiology and Biochemistry*, by kind permission of the author and Edward Arnold, 1968).

Insulin lowers the concentration of free fatty acids in the blood by increasing the permeability of the cell membranes to the free fatty acids and by inhibiting the break-down of triglycerides. The blood concentration of amino acids is also lowered by increasing the cell membrane permeability to amino acids and by direct action on some stage of protein synthesis (Fig.5.12).

In very general terms, insulin increases the permeability of cell membranes to small organic molecules (glucose, fatty acids, and amino acids), and stimulates the intracellular synthesis from those molecules to larger units.

Glucagon

The main supply of glucagon comes from the alpha-cells of the pancreas, but smaller amounts may be secreted by the mucosa of the stomach and the upper small intestine.

Unlike insulin, glucagon appears to act only intracellularly and not on the cell membrane. It stimulates the break-down of glycogen, protein, and triglycerides. It stimulates gluconeogenesis by the liver from the products of glycolysis and proteolysis. The stimulation of glycogen break-down is confined to the liver and does not apply to the skeletal muscle.

In general terms, the action of glucagon is to stimulate the catabolism of all three major classes of organic material. It raises plasma concentrations of glucose, non-esterified fatty acids and amino-acids.

REGULATION OF BLOOD GLUCOSE

Even in the absence of hormones, the blood glucose may be relatively steady provided that the animal is not subjected to starvation, excessive exercise or any other stress.

When the pancreas is removed in an animal the blood glucose rises rapidly, sugar appears in the urine and death soon follows. If the pituitary gland is removed as well, the control of blood glucose is much better, and the animal survives much longer. Under these circumstances, the blood glucose level depends primarily on the reaction between glucose and glucose-6-phosphate within the liver cells.

At a certain glucose concentration the rate of formation of glucose-6-phosphate from glucose and ATP will equal the rate of breakdown of glucose-6-phosphate to glucose and inorganic phosphate. An increase in blood glucose will speed up reaction (1) and slow down reaction (2) (Fig. 5.13). A fall in blood glucose will have the reverse effects. The glucose level will, therefore, tend to stay at the equilibrium position.

In order to ensure a stable blood glucose under changing conditions, hormonal control is essential. Two hormones, insulin and growth hormone, are primarily involved. Glucagon, cortisol, and adrenalin play a part in stress conditions.

The blood glucose level is lowered by insulin. The hormone increases glucose uptake and glycogen synthesis by the peripheral tissues (a), and it increases glycogen synthesis and decreases glucose outflow by the liver (b) (Fig.5.13).

The glucose level is raised by growth hormone, which breaks

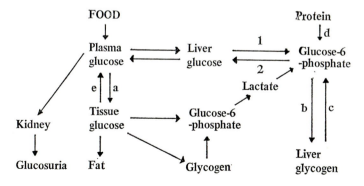

Fig.5.13. Summary of glucose metabolism (see text).

down triglycerides to supply free fatty acids and stimulates the metabolism of free fatty acids in preference to glucose. Blood glucose is also raised by glucagon, which increases liver glycogenolysis (c). When exposed to severe stress, the animal releases adrenalin which increases the liver glycogenolysis (c), and decreases the uptake of glucose by the partly permeable cells (e). ACTH stimulates the production of cortisol, which increases blood glucose by converting protein into glucose (d) (Fig. 5.13).

6

Food of domestic animals

The function of food is replacement of tissue in mature animals and building of tissue in young and pregnant animals. Food for animals comes from plants, directly in the case of herbivorous animals and indirectly in the case of carnivorous animals. From the soil the plant takes in water and salts, and from the atmosphere takes carbon dioxide and solar energy. All these substances and energy sources are the raw materials out of which it builds carbohydrates, fats, proteins, and other complex substances. The plant materials are then used by the animals with varying degrees of efficiency. Ruminants have the greatest capacity to utilize plant material—in particular cellulose-containing material—other herbivores less so, and carnivores least. From the proteins, fats, and carbohydrates the animal can derive energy and given the appropriate minerals and vitamins, can grow and reproduce.

ENERGY

For production, energy input must exceed energy output. The requirement for maintenance is the amount of energy the animal must expend on the various processes and reactions which are essential to life. The production requirement is the amount of energy which is needed in addition so that it may support the production of milk, eggs, meat, or fat, or meet the energy lost to the body in muscular work.

Energy inputs and outputs are measured in terms of calories, one cal being the amount of heat required to raise the temperature of 1 g of water 1 °C. The unit kilocalorie (kcal) is preferred. It represents the amount of heat required to raise the temperature of 1 kg of water through 1 °C.

The gross energy of a feed is the amount of heat liberated when it is burnt completely in a bomb calorimeter, the carbon and hydrogen in it being completely oxidized to CO_2 and H_2O. Gross energy values only state what energy the food contains not what the animal can obtain from it. Obviously only such parts of the food which can be digested by the animal furnish it with any useful energy. Most of what appears in the faeces has not been digested, and other substances are excreted by the body before they have been completely oxidized. Thus the nitrogen excreted in the urine is in the form of urea, hippuric acid and ammonia, and this excretion means a loss of energy. In the ruminants the production of combustible gases, mainly methane, also means a loss of energy.

The metabolizable energy is the gross energy, less the sum of the heat of the combustion of the faeces, fermentation gases, and urine. When intestinal fermentation is negligible, the metabolizable energy can be taken as the absorbed energy less the energy in the urine. Not all the metabolizable energy can be used by the animal for productive purposes nor for meeting its maintenance requirement, as a portion is always lost as heat. This is because a great deal of internal work must be done as in prehension, mastication, digestion, and assimilation. There is a further wastage of energy in the transference of absorbed nutrients to the tissues. The energy expended in the work of digestion and the losses entailed in metabolic transformations of the metabolizable energy are eventually given up as heat which may be of value under certain conditions for keeping the animal warm, but in general this heat is a waste product and in very hot climates it may even cause the animals to reduce their dry matter intake.

The net energy of the food is the energy which the animal actually uses for maintenance of its vital processes and for growth, deposition of fat and protein in its body, for production of its foetus, and for milk production. Net energy is thus metabolizable energy less heat production. The net energy of a feed may become negative if the metabolizable energy it supplies is less than the expenditure involved in its utilization. Straw has very little value for ruminants, and for horses it is worse than useless, since the horse expends more energy in eating and digesting it than the straw yields in metabolizable form.

CARBOHYDRATES

The carbohydrates of feeding stuffs include sugars, starch, cellulose, gums, and similar substances. As the complexity of these substances

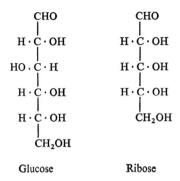

Fig.6.1. The formulae of glucose, a typical hexose monosaccharide, and of ribose, a typical pentose monosaccharide (Horrobin).

increases, the ease of digestion decreases. Cellulose, the principal structural carbohydrate, is the main constituent of crude fibre in plants. Feeds that contain a high percentage of cellulose, such as hay, silage, and straw, are called roughages and have a low digestibility. Seeds of plants and most of their by-products are quite low in cellulose. They are much more easily digestible and are known as concentrates.

The carbohydrates of animal feeds are generally classified according to their complexity as:

Monosaccharides are simple 5- or 6-carbon sugars, with the general formula $C_5H_{10}O_5$ for the pentoses, e.g. arabinose, xylose and ribose, and $C_6H_{12}O_6$ for the hexoses, e.g. glucose, fructose, galactose and mannose.

Disaccharides, consisting of two hexoses with the general formula $C_{12}H_{22}O_{11}$ which include sucrose, maltose, lactose, and cellobiose.

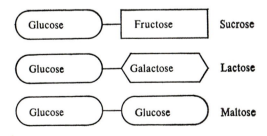

Fig.6.2. The constitution of the disaccharides, sucrose, lactose and maltose (Horrobin).

Polysaccharides are all of high molecular weight and are made up of condensations of simple sugars. They include the starches which are the main reserve carbohydrate in plants, and the dextrins which arise during the breakdown of starch. In the pig nearly all of the starches, dextrins, and disaccharides are hydrolyzed to simple sugars by enzymes secreted in the digestive tract. These simple sugars are then absorbed. The pectins, cellulose, lignin, hemicellulose, and pentosans are all cell wall carbohydrates. Cellulose and lignin are the most important of these, and they are the most abundant organic substances in the world. However, none of the enzymes secreted into the digestive tract of higher animals can carry out the hydrolysis of these compounds. For their digestion to occur microbial action is necessary.

In simple stomached animals little microbial fermentation occurs until the food residues reach the caecum and colon. In animals such as ruminants with a complex or multi-chambered stomach, great microbial activity is normal and there cellulose is attacked by bacteria to produce volatile fatty acids (VFA), acetic, propionic, and butyric acids. In the horse the large intestine is the main organ for microbial activity.

PROTEINS AND AMINO ACIDS

Proteins are complex, high molecular weight molecules made up primarily of amino acids. They contain carbon, hydrogen, oxygen, nitrogen, and usually sulphur. Some proteins contain phosphorus and iron. The functions of proteins are diverse and many. All of the known enzymes, many hormones, the oxygen carrying pigment of the blood and antibodies, are proteins.

Table 6.1 The percentage composition of common proteins

Nitrogen	Carbon	Oxygen	Hydrogen	Sulphur	Phosphorus
15–17	50–55	18–28	6·5–7·3	0·4–2·5	0·1

Proteins are composed of chains of amino acids. Their molecular weights may range from 6000 in a simple molecule like insulin to many millions in the complex proteins of a virus particle. The simple proteins yield only amino acids upon hydrolysis. Included in the simple proteins are albumins, globulins, and glutelins. The conjugated proteins consist of simple proteins combined with a non protein radical. Examples of these include nucleoproteins (protein + nucleic acid), glycoproteins (proteins + carbohydrate group), and phosphoproteins (protein + phosphorous containing group). The derived proteins are breakdown products of naturally occurring proteins.

The amino acids consist largely of carbon, hydrogen and oxygen. They are characterized by having a carboxyl group ($-COOH$) and an amino group ($-NH_2$) attached to the same carbon atom. Also attached to this same alpha-carbon atom is another carbon-hydrogen group designated R

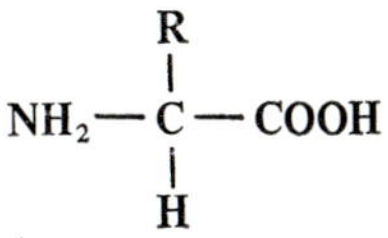

$$NH_2 - \overset{\displaystyle R}{\underset{\displaystyle H}{C}} - COOH$$

Fig.6.3. The general structure of the alpha-amino acid molecule.

The amino acids which cannot be synthesized in the non-ruminant or calf in its pre-ruminant stage, or at a rate adequate to meet the needs for growth and reproduction, are termed essential amino acids and must be present in the diet. Those which the non-ruminant or calf in the pre-ruminant stage can synthesize at adequate rates from the other nitrogenous sources are termed non-essential. In the case of ruminants, microbial synthesis can largely overcome the need for preformed protein or essential amino acids in the food since the bacteria can synthesize the protein from non-protein non-amino acid sources in sufficient amounts. The microbial protein is subsequently digested and the liberated amino acids supply all those essential for growth and production.

The essential amino acids are: lysine, tryptophan, histidine, phenylalanine, leucine, isoleucine, threonine, methionine, valine, and arginine. The non-essential amino acids are: glycine, alanine, serine, cysteine, tyrosine, aspartic acid, glutamic acid, proline, hydroxyproline, and citrulline.

Deficiency in an essential amino acid leads to failure in growth and may lead eventually to death. In general, animal proteins, such as those of blood meal, meat and bone meal, and fish meal are much superior to plant proteins as sources of essential amino acids. But it is possible to supplement plant proteins or have them in such an

3

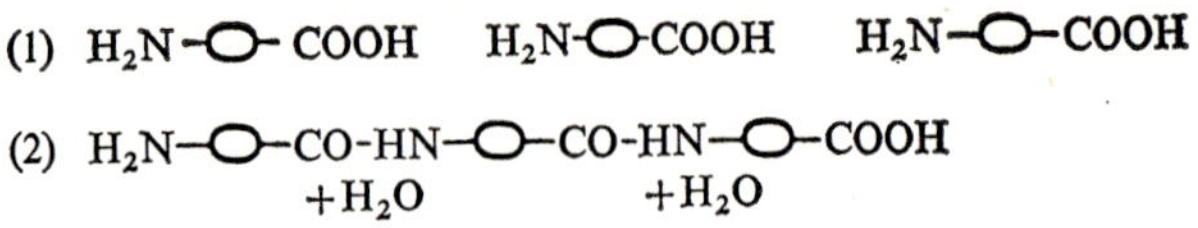

(1) $H_2N-\bigcirc-COOH$ $H_2N-\bigcirc-COOH$ $H_2N-\bigcirc-COOH$

(2) $H_2N-\bigcirc-CO-HN-\bigcirc-CO-HN-\bigcirc-COOH$
$\quad\quad\quad\quad +H_2O \quad\quad\quad\quad +H_2O$

Fig.6.4. The linking of amino acids to form a protein. (1) Shows three separate amino acids. (2) Shows the three linked together by peptide bonds (Horrobin).

admixture that their individual deficiencies are compensated by the pattern of amino acids in the rest of the feed.

The amino acids of proteins are joined one to the other by a peptide bond, a union between the amino group of one acid and the carboxyl group of another acid, with the elimination of a molecule of water.

LIPIDS

The lipids are characterized by their sparing solubility in water and their considerable solubility in organic solvents. They are classified as simple and compound lipids. Simple lipids, which are esters of fatty acids and alcohols, and

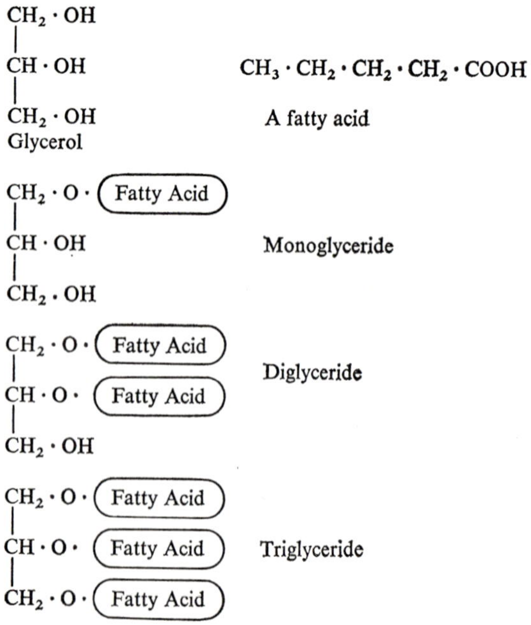

$$CH_2 \cdot OH$$
$$|$$
$$CH \cdot OH \quad\quad\quad\quad\quad CH_3 \cdot CH_2 \cdot CH_2 \cdot CH_2 \cdot COOH$$
$$|$$
$$CH_2 \cdot OH \quad\quad\quad\quad\quad \text{A fatty acid}$$
Glycerol

$$CH_2 \cdot O \cdot \boxed{\text{Fatty Acid}}$$
$$|$$
$$CH \cdot OH \quad\quad\quad\quad \text{Monoglyceride}$$
$$|$$
$$CH_2 \cdot OH$$

$$CH_2 \cdot O \cdot \boxed{\text{Fatty Acid}}$$
$$|\quad\quad\quad\quad\quad\quad\quad \text{Diglyceride}$$
$$CH \cdot O \cdot \boxed{\text{Fatty Acid}}$$
$$|$$
$$CH_2 \cdot OH$$

$$CH_2 \cdot O \cdot \boxed{\text{Fatty Acid}}$$
$$|$$
$$CH \cdot O \cdot \boxed{\text{Fatty Acid}} \quad\quad \text{Triglyceride}$$
$$|$$
$$CH_2 \cdot O \cdot \boxed{\text{Fatty Acid}}$$

Fig.6.5. The formulae of glycerol, a fatty acid, and the various types of glyceride (Horrobin).

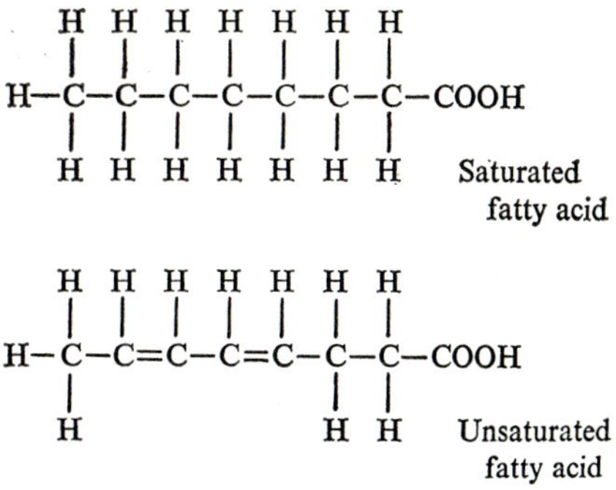

Fig.6.6. Formulae of a saturated and an unsaturated fatty acid to show the difference between the two (Horrobin).

include fats (esters of fatty acids and glycerol) and waxes (esters of fatty acids and alcohols other than glycerol). Compound lipids contain some other group besides alcohol and fatty acid, such as phosphoric acid, nitrogen, or carbohydrate. Derived lipids are compounds resulting from hydrolysis of simple or compound lipids.

In general the fats (glycerides) have a much greater feeding value than the non glycerides, but the latter include vitamins A, D, E and K, which are essential nutrients.

The saturated fatty acids have twice as many hydrogen atoms as carbon atoms, and each molecule of fatty acid contains two atoms of oxygen. Examples of saturated fatty acids are: butyric acid $CH_3CH_2CH_2COOH$ and palmitic acid $CH_3(CH_2)_{14}COOH$. Saturated fatty acids with up to 6 carbon atoms are liquids, whereas acids with more than 6 carbon atoms are solids at normal room temperatures. The unsaturated fatty acids contain less than twice as many hydrogen atoms as carbon atoms, and one or more pairs of adjacent atoms are connected by double bonds. An example of an unsaturated fatty acid is oleic acid $CH_3(CH_2)_7CH=CH(CH_2)7COOH$ (Fig. 6.6).

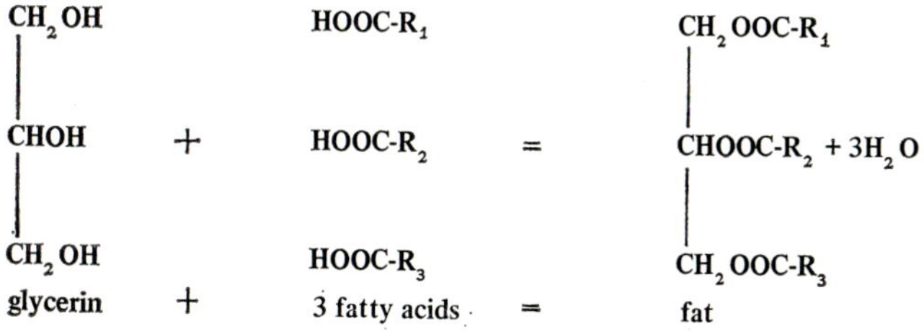

Fig.6.7. The principal structure of a natural fat. R–COOH is used as the formula for any fatty acid.

Natural fat is an ester of three molecules of fatty acids (all may be the same or may be different acids) combined with one molecule of glycerol (Fig.6.7).

MINERALS

The ash constituents of a feeding stuff or animal tissue are determined by incinerating the dry material to constant weight. The remaining material is extracted with hot diluted acid and filtered. The major minerals in relation to animals are calcium, phosphorus, potassium, sodium, chloride, and magnesium. These elements are all of nutritional significance. Of the other main mineral elements found in plants little is known, but it is generally accepted that they are not essential to animals. There are, however, a number of minerals which are essential to animals in trace amounts. Given in excess some of these elements produce toxic effects. The trace mineral elements required by higher animals are: iron, copper, molybdenum, cobalt, zinc, and manganese, and amongst the non-metals: iodine, fluorine, and selenium.

Though deficiency or excess of certain trace elements can cause bad health or even death, much more harm to the productivity of domestic animals is generally done by shortage of the essential major minerals in their daily rations. The deficiency of a mineral may arise in several ways. The soil may be deficient in a particular mineral or the mineral may be present but unavailable to the plants eaten by the animals. In either case the plant itself fails to grow if the mineral is essential to it, or if it does grow, it becomes deficient in this particular element. It may also be that the diet contains an adequate supply of minerals but if one or more of them is in an unavailable form the animals will not thrive.

Sodium

Most animal protein concentrates are rich in sodium (0·5–1 per cent) of fresh weight), whereas protein concentrates derived from vegetable sources contain appreciably less (0·05–0·3 per cent). The sodium content of fresh grass varies (0·02–0·25 per cent) and is markedly depressed when the potassium level of the soil is increased. In dairy cows at the peak of lactation the supply of sodium from grass may be insufficient to meet requirements if the content of this element is less than 0·04 per cent.

Sodium is concerned with maintaining the osmotic pressure in the extracellular fluid and thereby regulating the body fluid volume. It also plays an important role in nerve impulse transmission in which the development of the action potential is associated with a sudden influx of the sodium ion. Diets low in sodium or excessive losses of this element in sweat or in urine may lead to sufficient depletion to lower the concentration of sodium in the extracellular fluid compartment with the result that water may be transferred from this compartment to tissue cells to restore osmotic equilibrium. The cells will become over-hydrated; the degree of such a hydration is a function of both sodium and water losses.

The sodium requirement of growing pigs increases from 0·4 to 1·0 g per day as the live weight increases from 5 kg to 90 kg. Dry cows require approximately 8 g per day, and cows in full lactation up to 20 g per day. The requirement for sheep is about 1 g per day.

Chloride

Chloride occurs in the food together with sodium. Its major function in the animal body is shared with the sodium ion in maintaining the osmotic pressure of extracellular fluids. Being the major anion in the extracellular fluid together with bicarbonate, chloride is of importance in maintaining electroneutrality in cases of changes in the acid-base balance. Another important function of chloride is in the production of hydrochloric acid in the stomach.

The chloride requirement of growing cattle gaining weight at about 0·5 kg/day rises from 1·8 to 10·9 g/day as the live weight increases from 50 to 400 kg. The chloride requirement for growing sheep is within the range 0·35–1·6 g/day increasing with live weight and rate of growth.

Potassium

Vegetable protein concentrates are rich in potassium (1–2 per cent of the fresh weight). The potassium content of grass is markedly influenced by the level of potassium fertilization. The potassium : sodium ratio in crops fertilized with potash fertilizers may rise to 50 : 1. Whole cereal grain and most vegetable crops contain between 0·1 and 0·5 per cent. The high potassium content in many feeding stuffs and the fact that the greater part of the element in these materials appears to be in a freely soluble ionic form of high availability are responsible for the fact that potassium deficiency arising from an inadequate intake is unknown.

Potassium is present in high concentrations within most tissue cells. It is of importance for maintaining the osmotic pressure in the intracellular fluid space and for the normal function of the nervous and muscular systems. The potassium ion is furthermore an enzyme activator for the transphosphorylation of phosphate from pyruvate-enolphosphate to ADP, and is thus of importance for the metabolism of carbohydrates.

Calcium

Roughages such as lucerne, grass, and hay are rich in calcium, and so are the animal concentrates, meat and bone meal and fish meal. The main part of the body calcium (99 per cent) is found in the skeleton as phosphates and carbonates bound in a complex. Part of the bone calcium is labile and in equilibrium with the ionized calcium in the plasma. Blood plasma contains 9–11 mg calcium per 100 ml blood, half of which is present as ionized calcium, the rest bound to plasma albumin. Change in the pH of the blood alters the ratio between ionized and protein bound calcium. If the pH falls (acidosis) the amount of ionized calcium increases, and if the pH rises (alkalosis) ionized calcium decreases.

In the lactating animal large amounts of calcium are excreted in the milk. In cows the calcium concentration in the blood falls 1–1·5 mg per 100 ml following milking. Calcium concentrations below 5 mg/100 ml leads to milk fever.

Calcium is of importance for the normal development of the skeleton and for the normal function of the cardiac and skeletal muscles. The calcium ion is also of importance as an enzyme activator for lipase and thrombokinase.

Phosphorus

Feeding stuffs of animal origin have the highest contents of phosphorus, usually in a highly available form. Among common feeding stuffs, fish meal and meat and bone meal are by far the richest sources. The cereal grains usually contain 0·3–0·4 per cent phosphorus, whereas most cereal straws are extremely low in phosphorus.

Between 20 and 25 per cent of the phosphorus in the body is present in the extraskeletal soft tissue in contrast to calcium where only 1 per cent is found in tissues other than bone. Some of the phosphorus in soft tissue may be regarded as having structural function, e.g. the phospholipids of the central nervous system, but the greater part is present in phosphate-containing metabolic intermediates in the synthesis and degradation of carbohydrates, proteins and nucleic acids.

In non-ruminants it has been shown that increasing the calcium : phosphorus ratio of the diet may interfere with the absorption of phosphorus and, conversely, that a high phosphorus to calcium ratio may restrict calcium absorption. The magnitude of this effect differs between species, depends upon the forms of calcium and phosphorus present in the diet, and also upon the vitamin D status of the animal, the effect being greater when the vitamin D intake is low.

In growing pigs, changes in the calcium : phosphorus ratio from 1 : 1 to 2 : 1 show little if any effect on calcium and phosphorus utilization, whereas ratios over 2 : 1 may adversely affect phosphorus utilization, particularly if the phosphorus content in the diet is below 0·4 per cent.

In growing chicks the optimum ratio is between 1·5 : 1 and 2 : 1 when calculated on the basis of available phosphorus.

Growing ruminants appear to be less sensitive to changes in the calcium : phosphorus ratio, and this has to be increased to 8 : 1 before an adverse effect on performance is apparent. Despite this wider tolerance by ruminants, recognition of the facts that the ratio of these elements in the body is about 1·8 : 1 and in milk approximately 1·3 or 1·4 : 1 makes it desirable to ensure that the available calcium : phosphorus ratio in all ruminant rations is maintained within the ranges 1 : 1 or 2 : 1, particularly in rapidly growing and heavy-milking animals.

In young animals deficiency in calcium and phosphorus causes softening of the bones and therefore malformations, a disease known as rickets. In the adult animal lack of calcium and phosphorus causes weakening of the bones and frequent fractures—osteomalacia.

In cattle the dietary calcium requirement is a function of rate of growth or stage of pregnancy or lactation. For a 100 kg animal the requirement is nearly trebled by increasing the rate of gain from 0·3–1·0 kg per day, the estimated needs for calcium being 11 and 27 g per day. Under the same circumstances the phosphorus requirement increases from 5–13 g per day respectively. The effects of lactation are even more striking, the calcium requirement of a 500 kg cow increasing from 30 g per day when producing 5 kg of milk per day to 100 g per day when producing 30 kg. Pigs require 12–15 g calcium and 8 to 10 g phosphorus per day for maintenance, and 6–8 g of calcium and 3–5 g of phosphorus per day during pregnancy. In addition to maintenance, 30 g calcium and 20 g phosphorus per day is necessary for production of milk for a litter of 8–10 pigs.

Magnesium

All natural feedstuffs contain magnesium. The vegetable protein concentrates usually contain large amounts, 0·4–0·6 per cent of the dry matter. Also grass and clovers are rich in magnesium. Of the concentrates, bran has a high magnesium content.

Between 50 and 75 per cent of the total body magnesium is found in the skeleton where the normal calcium : magnesium ratio is about 55 : 1. A large proportion of the skeletal magnesium is not readily exchangeable with magnesium in the tissue fluids. Between 15 and 50 per cent of the total plasma magnesium is bound to serum proteins.

Magnesium plays a vital role as an activator of many enzymes which transfer and split phosphorus groups. It is also involved in enzymatic decarboxylations, in protein and peptide hydrolysis, and in protein synthesis. Hyperirritability and convulsions are typical signs of magnesium deficiency in all species of farm animals, indicating that magnesium has a role in the maintenance of normal nerve function. A role in muscular function is suggested by the muscular weakness that develops in the deficient animal. Magnesium deficiency in dairy cattle causes a disease known as grass tetany.

The magnesium requirement depends upon the physiological state of the animal. Thus the requirement of a 500 kg animal lies between 8 and 10 g per day depending on the rate of growth, whereas in the lactating cow of the same weight producing 20 kg of milk per day the requirement is as high as 20 g per day. In sheep the requirement varies between 0·5 and 1 g per day according to how fast the animal is growing.

Iron

Iron is found in all feeds, but mainly in grass and straw. Only about 5–20 per cent of the iron in the feed can be utilized by the animals. The animal body contains about 0·004 per cent iron of which 60 per cent is found in the haemoglobin of the erythrocytes, 3–5 per cent in the myoglobin of muscle, 7–15 per cent as the iron storage protein ferritin, 0·2 per cent in enzymes, and 0·1 per cent as beta-globulin transferrin in the plasma.

As a consequence of the low reserves of iron at birth and the low content of this element in milk, piglets are particularly dependent upon extraneous sources of supply to maintain haemoglobin production during early life. Iron deficiency causes anaemia. Effective control is achieved by either oral administration of ferrous salts or intramuscular injection of iron complexes.

Copper

All feedstuffs contain copper, but in varying amounts according to the concentration of copper in the soil. Much of the copper in the blood plasma is associated with alpha-globulin. The remainder of the plasma copper is loosely bound to albumin and it is this fraction which initially rises following copper uptake. Certain organs, particularly the liver, kidney, heart, and spleen, have high concentrations of copper relative to other tissues.

The element plays an important role in the respiratory enzyme cytochrome oxidase, and in the formation of the porphyrin nucleus of the haemoglobin molecule. Copper deficiency is more common in ruminants than in non-ruminants, arising either from a low copper intake or from the presence in the diet of factors which interfere with copper utilization. The typical picture of copper deficiency in cattle is one of poor growth, anaemia, bone fragility and sometimes diarrhoea. In sheep the signs of depressed growth rate and anaemia are rare. Instead, the most significant effects are during late foetal and early post-natal development in lamb where copper deficiency causes degenerative changes in nervous tissue, leading to blindness, incoordination of the hind limbs, and progressing immobilization.

In pigs it has been found that 6 p.p.m. (parts per million) copper in the ration allows normal growth and haemoglobin production. In ruminants the copper requirements are less well defined because of the uncertainties of the nature of dietary components which can decrease availability. It seems however that deficiency may be expected in cattle and sheep when the copper content of pasture falls below 4 p.p.m.

Cobalt

Cobalt in trace quantities is widely distributed in common feedstuffs. As mentioned for copper the amount of cobalt in plants depends on the cobalt content of the soil where the plant is grown.

The only functional form of tissue cobalt is as part of vitamin B_{12}. In addition to the roles of this vitamin in transmethylation, erythropoesis and purine biosynthesis, its role in tissue propionate metabolism is of particular importance to the ruminant which depends upon propionate produced in the rumen for a large part of its energy requirements. Vitamin B_{12} is necessary to convert propionate into succinate which is an intermediate in the tricarboxylic acid cycle.

Ruminants deficient in cobalt show emaciation and anorexia and in later stages anaemia. The disease is common in areas where the concentration of cobalt in pasture falls below 0·08 p.p.m.

Table 6.2 Content of minerals in the animal body

Element	% of body weight	Amount in cow (500 kg)
Ca	2·0	10 000 g
P	1·2	6000 g
K	0·35	1800 g
S	0·25	1250 g
Na	0·15	750 g
Cl	0·15	750 g
Mg	0·06	300 g
Fe	0·004	20 g
Zn	0·002	10 g
Cu	0·000 15	750 mg
Mn	0·000 13	650 mg

VITAMINS

Vitamins are organic compounds necessary in small quantities to ensure normal growth. They act in the organism as parts of enzyme systems and deficiencies cause characteristic diseases in animals. Under practical conditions it is unusual to see deficiency of only one vitamin; an inadequate diet will often lack several vitamins.

The minimum requirement of a given vitamin is the amount that is necessary to prevent disease, whereas the maximum requirement is the amount that secures maximum growth, fertility, milk production etc.

The vitamins are divided into two groups on the basis of their solubility. The fat soluble vitamins are either soluble in fat or absorbed with fat. They are vitamins A, D, E and K. The water soluble vitamins are either soluble in water or absorbed with water. They are vitamins B and C.

Vitamin A

Vitamin A is only found in feeds of animal origin. In plants, pro-

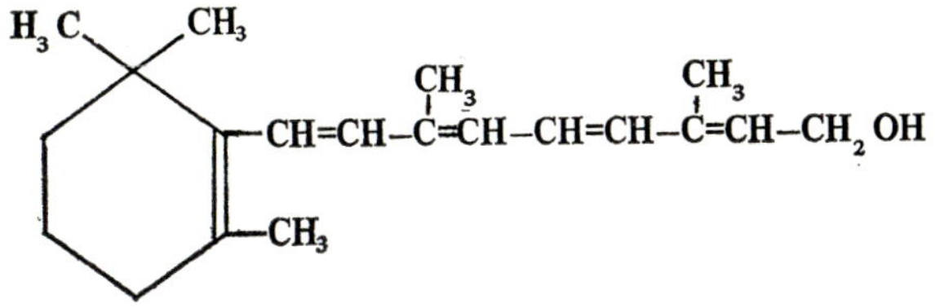

Fig.6.8. The chemical configuration of vitamin A.

vitamins or precursors for the vitamin are found, known as alpha-, beta-, and gamma-carotene. The pro-vitamins are converted to vitamin A in the intestinal mucosa during absorption.

The biochemical functions of vitamin A in the animal body are not known in detail. The vitamin is important for normal growth and for normal function of the epithelial tissues. An important sign of vitamin A deficiency is inability to see at low light intensity, due to the role of vitamin A in the synthesis of rhodopsin. Vitamin A deficiency in chicken causes incoordination of movements, slow growth rate, and high mortality. In hens the eyes become swollen and egg production falls. Sows fed a diet insufficient in the vitamin give birth to blind and malformed pigs. Cows suffering from vitamin A deficiency develop anoestrus (do not come into heat). Calves are often born weak or dead.

Vitamin D

Vitamin D is found in two forms, D_2 and D_3. Vitamin D_2 is formed by solar radiation of the pro-vitamin ergosterol found in yeast, grass, and lucerne. Vitamin D_3 is formed by solar radiation of the pro-vitamin 7-dehydrocholesterol, which is found in the skin of mammals.

In mammals vitamins D_2 and D_3 have the same biological effect, whereas in fowl the effect of D_3 is 50 to 100 times that of D_2. Under natural conditions the animals synthesize vitamin D using solar radiation of their skin. The vitamin is partly absorbed through the skin, partly obtained by licking. Omnivorous and carnivorous animals get their vitamin D supply partly or completely from feed of animal origin. In suckling animals the vitamin is supplied by the milk.

Vitamin D stimulates the absorption rate of calcium and phosphorus in the intestinal tract, and thereby aids the development of

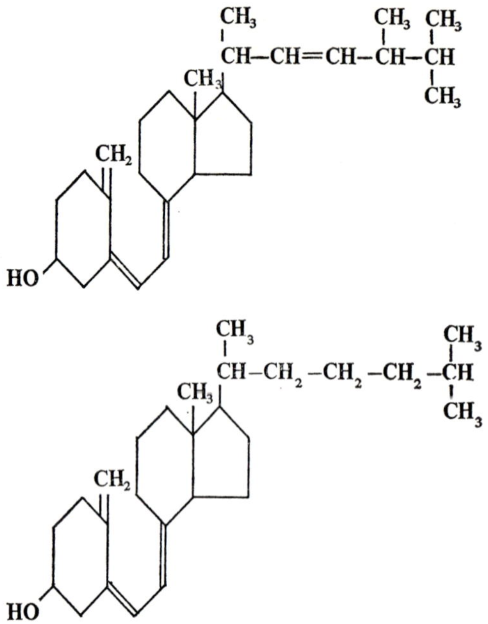

Fig.6.9. The chemical configuration of vitamins D_2 and D_3.

bones, teeth, and the thickness of the eggshell. The vitamin also regulates the deposition of calcium and phosphorus in the bones, and stimulates the reabsorption of phosphorus in the kidney tubules.

The symptoms of vitamin D deficiency in chickens are lameness, paralysis, swollen joints, and malformation of bones, especially the sternum. In pigs deficiency in the vitamin causes malformation of the bones and a high frequency of fractures. In cows there is suppression of the milk production.

Table 6.3 Daily requirements of vitamins A and D. Values represent maximal requirements. (For ruminants 1 mg carotene = 125 international units (i.u.) vitamin A, for pigs 1 mg carotene = 200 i.u.)

Animal	mg carotene	i.u. vit. A	i.u. vit. D
Calves	40	5000	500
Young cattle	40–120	15 000	1000
Cows (milking)	240	30 000	3000
Sheep and goats	30	4000	400
Young pigs	15	3000	300
Sows	50	10 000	1000

Vitamin E

Vitamin E, tocopherol, is necessary for normal reproduction in some animals. The vitamin is mainly found in grass, lucerne, and wheat bran. Deficiency over a prolonged period leads to degeneration of skeletal and heart muscle.

In chicken, deficiency leads to degeneration of the brain and uncontrolled movements (crazy chick disease) and in hens to sterility. In pigs lack of the vitamin causes abnormal colour of the fat and fetal death. In lambs the effect on the muscles is most pronounced leading to a disease known as stiff lamb disease.

Vitamin K

Vitamin K is necessary for the formation of prothrombin, a substance essential to blood clotting. The vitamin is formed by microorganisms in the digestive tract, and is also found in green plants and fish meal.

Certain plants contain a compound, coumarin, which can be changed to dicoumarol by intestinal micro-organisms. The structure of the dicoumarol molecule is like the structure of the vitamin K molecule, but without its effect. When an animal absorbs large amounts of dicoumarol, this compound will replace vitamin K and a vitamin deficiency will develop resulting in internal haemorrages because of the failure of the blood to clot.

Dicoumarol is used as an effective rat poison, and precautions must be taken to ensure that the poison does not reach domestic animals.

Vitamin B$_1$

Vitamin B$_1$ or thiamine is found in most feedstuffs. The vitamin is of importance in carbohydrate metabolism in that it acts as an enzyme for the oxidative decarboxylation of pyruvic acid to acetyl-CoA.

Deficiency of thiamine causes beriberi in man and polyneuritis in birds. Ruminants and most other mammals do not ordinarily need additional thiamine in the diet because micro-organisms in the digestive tract synthesize more thiamine than needed by the host animal.

In chicken, lack of the vitamin causes polyneuritis (inflammation of the nerves), lack of appetite, and stiff neck muscles.

Vitamin B_2

Vitamin B_2 or riboflavin is found in most feedstuffs, but mainly in milk and lucerne. It is synthesized in sufficient amounts by the intestinal microflora.

The vitamin is important as co-enzyme in oxidation processes. Deficiency symptoms in chickens include slow growth rate, weak legs and paralysed toes. Hens lay few eggs and the chicks are often malformed. In pigs, lack of riboflavin causes stiffness of muscles, diarrhoea, and eczema. In sows there is premature birth and the piglets are weak.

Niacin

This vitamin is found in most feeds and is produced in the intestinal tract from the amino acid tryptophan. When maize is fed, niacin deficiency may occur owing to lack of tryptophan. The vitamin forms the active group in co-enzyme I and II (DPN and TPN).

Lack of the vitamin causes loss of appetite and low utilization of food in pigs.

Vitamin B_6

Vitamin B_6 or pyridoxine is important to ensure normal growth and protein synthesis in animals. It is also of importance in the synthesis of haemoglobin.

Lack of the vitamin causes anaemia, loss of appetite, and low utilization of protein.

Pantothenic acid

Pantothenic acid is found in all feedstuffs but in varying amounts. Bran and lucerne are rich in the vitamin whereas meat and bone meal only contain small amounts. Pantothenic acid forms part of co-enzyme A, which acts in the transfer of acetyl groups. It is of importance for the synthesis of acetylcholine, fatty acids, and some amino acids.

Deficiency of the vitamin leads to dermatitis, loss of hair, graying of hair, and lesions of various organs.

Vitamin B_{12}

Vitamin B_{12} or cobalamin is a vitamin containing cobalt (see page 61).

Vitamin C

Vitamin C or ascorbic acid is synthesized by most animals. Guinea pigs, monkeys, and man, however, must receive their ascorbic acid in the diet. Deficiency of the vitamin causes scurvy, the symptoms of which are bleeding of the gums and damage to the teeth.

Table 6.4 Daily requirement of vitamin B for pigs

Vitamin	µg per kg body weight
Thiamine	75
Riboflavin	60
Niacin	250
Pantothenic acid	500
Pyridoxine	100

7

Digestion in simple stomached animals

MOUTH AND PHARYNX

In all animals the food is brought into the mouth by means of lips, teeth and tongue. The lips of the horse, the tongue of the cow and sheep and the snout of the pig are used extensively in obtaining food. Fluid is obtained differently in different animals. Horses, ruminants and pigs drink by suction. The lips are kept closed except for the part kept under the surface and a vacuum is created in the mouth by the tongue. Carnivorous animals drink by licking. Suckling animals drink by creating an extensive vacuum in the mouth. A new born calf will suckle 10–16 times per day and drink 300–400 ml of milk each time. New born pigs suckle 14–20 times per day, taking 40–60 ml each time.

Mastication, or chewing, differs in various animals. Carnivorous animals have simple teeth and tear their food but do little grinding. In herbivorous animals mastication is of major importance and food is thoroughly ground between the molar teeth. Mastication in pigs resembles that of carnivorous animals.

During mastication the food is mixed with saliva. The secretion of saliva is an intermittent process commencing after several chewing movements. The stimulus comes from receptors in the mouth. The glands receive parasympathetic and sympathetic nerve fibres. Stimulation of the parasympathetic fibres increases the blood supply to the glands and causes secretion of generous amounts of rather thin saliva. Sympathetic stimulation decreases blood supply and either inhibits flow of saliva or causes secretion of a thick mucous type of saliva.

The daily secretion varies with the kind of food eaten. Dry food causes watery and copious saliva, whereas moist food reduces the volume. The average volume secreted amounts to about 15 litres per 24 hours in pigs and 40–50 litres per 24 hours in horses.

The formation of secretion varies; some compounds are found in the same or lower concentration as in the extracellular fluid and they are secreted by simple diffusion or by filtration. Other compounds are found in higher concentration in the saliva than in the extracellular fluid and must be secreted by an active process. Finally some compounds are found entirely in the saliva and must be formed by the cells of the gland from compounds in the blood.

In the simple stomached animals saliva has a pH of 6·8–7·4, in ruminants saliva is alkaline with a pH between 8·1 and 8·8. This is caused by the high concentration of bicarbonate and phosphate that makes ruminant saliva a rather highly concentrated bicarbonate–phosphate buffer solution. The parotid gland produces a serous alkaline fluid which in pigs, but not in horses, contains small amounts of the enzyme amylase. This enzyme catalyzes the hydrolysis of starch. The amylase activity of pig saliva is many times less than that found in humans. The secretion from the other salivary glands contains no enzymes. It is a water-clear, slimy, slightly alkaline fluid that moistens the food to facilitate swallowing and further enzyme action.

The act of swallowing is arbitrarily divided into three stages. The first stage is under voluntary control. After the food has been chewed and mixed with saliva a bolus is formed, which is placed on the upper surface of the tongue. The tongue is then raised against the hard palate, moving the bolus towards the pharynx. At the same time the soft palate is raised, closing the posterior nares, and the base of the tongue forces the bolus into the pharynx.

As the bolus enters the pharynx it touches sensitive areas which reflexly initiate the second stage, the passage of the bolus through the pharynx. Respiration is reflexly inhibited, and the larynx closed. The pharynx is shortened and a peristaltic action of the pharyngeal muscles forces the bolus into the oesophagus.

The third stage consists of a reflex peristalsis of the oesophagus initiated by the pressure of the food in the oesophagus. Solid food is carried to the stomach at a speed of 30–40 cm per second.

STOMACH

The simple stomached animals include carnivores, omnivores, and some herbivores. Since the type of food varies in these animals some

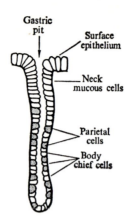

Fig.7.1. Outline of the structure of a gastric gland from the middle part of the stomach (from Horrobin, *Medical Physiology and Biochemistry*, by kind permission of the author and Edward Arnold, 1968).

difference is seen in the function of the stomach. The following is mainly based on the function of the stomach of the dog and the pig as little is known about the function of the stomach of the horse.

The stomach may be divided into three zones corresponding to three different types of mucosa. The oral part of the stomach, known as the cardia, contains mucous glands. These glands produce an alkaline mucous secretion which contains no enzymes. The secretion of the cardiac glands does not contribute very much to the total amount of gastric juice. The main function of this secretion is to protect the gastric mucosa against the hydrochloric acid secreted from the fundic glands.

The middle part of the stomach is the fundus and the fundus glands are the main contributors of gastric juice. These glands are long narrow tubules containing three types of cells—chief cells, parietal cells, and mucous neck cells (Fig.7.1). The chief cells are responsible for the secretion of enzymes (mainly pepsin), the parietal cells for the secretion of hydrochloric acid, and the neck cells for the production of mucus.

The aboral part of the stomach, the pylorus, contains glands that produce a mucous secretion.

The mixed gastric juice is composed of secretions from all three parts of the stomach. The cardia and pylorus secrete neutral or slightly alkaline juice, while the fundus secretes a very acid juice. The mixed juice contains both inorganic and organic matter. The organic matter is mainly the enzyme pepsin; the inorganic is NaCl,

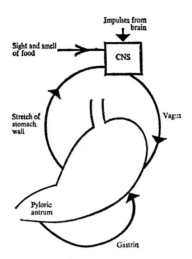

Impulses from brain

Sight and smell of food

CNS

Stretch of stomach wall

Vagus

Pyloric antrum

Gastrin

Fig.7.2. The control of gastric secretion (Horrobin).

KCl, $CaCl_2$, and $MgCl_2$. The parietal cells contain an enzyme, carbonic anhydrase, which catalyzes the process:

$$CO_2 + H_2O \rightarrow H_2CO_3 \rightarrow H^+ + HCO_3^-$$

The H^+ is excreted into the lumen of the stomach, the HCO_3^- is exchanged with Cl^- from the extracellular fluid, and the Cl^- is excreted. If the carbonic anhydrase is destroyed the production of HCl ceases.

The secretion of gastric juice is intermittent. In the fasting animal with an empty stomach practically no secretion takes place. The secretion is initiated as soon as the animal starts eating. This phase of gastric secretion is known as the nervous phase. It is controlled by afferent neurons from the taste buds in the mouth, and efferent neurons in the vagal nerve. The secretion begins 2–3 minutes after food has entered the mouth and continues for 1–2 hours.

If the food remains more than 1–2 hours in the stomach, the secretion continues. This demonstrates that the presence of food in the stomach stimulates gastric secretion. When the partly digested food reaches the pylorus, a chemical, gastrin, is released from the mucous membrane to the blood. Gastrin is carried by the blood to the fundus where it stimulates the cells to produce gastric juice (Fig. 7.2).

When the contents of the stomach are emptied into the duodenum the intestinal mucosa produces another hormone secretion which also stimulates the secretion of the fundic glands.

Feeding fat decreases the gastric secretion. Fat stimulates the duodenal mucosa to release to the blood a chemical, enterogastrone, that reaches the fundus via the blood and inhibits both HCl and pepsin secretion.

When the stomach is empty it is fully contracted. When it is full, steady tonic contractions run continuously with 2–3 waves each minute. The contractions originate in the cardiac region and progress towards the pylorus, causing the most digested food to reach the pylorus where peristaltic contractions mix it and send it into the duodenum. The material that leaves the stomach is called chyme. During the period of chyme evacuation, duodenal motility is inhibited. However, the duodenal wall resumes its tone and rhythmic activity approximately at the same time as the sphincter muscle contracts. Regurgitation of chyme from duodenum is prevented by the sphincter, whereas this structure plays no important part in the regulation or rate of gastric emptying.

Table 7.1 Gastrointestinal hormones

Origin	Hormone	Releasing mechanism	Function
Pylorus	Gastrin	Partly digested food in pylorus	Stimulation of acid secretion by gastric glands
Duodenum	Enterogastrone	Fat and fatty acids plus bile in duodenum	Inhibition of gastric secretion and motility
Duodenum	Secretin	Acid and peptones in duodenum	Stimulation of pancreatic secretion (water and electrolytes)
Duodenum	Pancreozymin	Acid and peptones in duodenum	Stimulation of pancreatic secretion (enzymes)
Duodenum	Cholecystokinin	Fat in duodenum	Contraction of gall bladder
Jejunum	Enterocrinin	Food digestion products	Stimulation of intestinal secretion

The stomach movements are regulated by the autonomic nervous system. Stimulation of the vagal nerve increases the motility and stimulation of the sympathetic nervous system inhibits motility.

Gastric emptying

The emptying of food from the stomach after a meal begins as soon as any considerable part of the gastric contents becomes fluid enough to pass through the pylorus. Once started, the emptying proceeds rhythmically, a small amount being evacuated at a time.

The rate of emptying is regulated by the accumulation of material from the stomach in the duodenum. Both the volume and the chemical composition of the duodenal contents are important in inhibiting gastric emptying. Effective chemical inhibitors include fat, fatty acids, peptides, amino acids, hydrogen ions and sugars and other products of starch digestion. The effect of these substances in the duodenum is to reduce the tone and peristaltic activity of the stomach muscles thus reducing the pressure gradient between stomach and duodenum which develops with each cycle of gastric contraction and which is responsible for the passage of fluid through the pylorus.

The inhibitory effect may be exerted in several different ways. The food in the duodenum excites both stretch and chemical receptors in the duodenal wall. Some of the impulses which are fired off by these receptors go to the central nervous system where they inhibit the activity of the vagal nerve which is responsible for stimulating gastric contractions. Other impulses pass directly along the plexuses in the gut wall and inhibit stomach activity that way. Stretch and chemical stimulation also cause the release of a hormone from the duodenal wall. This is known as enterogastrone and passes into the blood from the duodenal mucous membrane. It circulates to the stomach where it inhibits gastric contractions. Products of protein digestion, acids and non-specific irritants act mainly via the nerves while fats and carbohydrates act mainly through the hormone.

Digestive processes in the stomach

The stomach of carnivores will empty within a few hours after a meal, whereas horses and pigs require a full day's fast to empty a full stomach. Hence, when they eat there is still some material from the last meal left in the stomach and recently swallowed food will settle as a layer upon the contents already present in the stomach. The intimate mixing of the gastric contents first takes place in the pyloric region where the peristaltic waves running through the stomach wall are strongest.

Because of this slow mixing of the gastric contents it takes rather a long time before the food comes into contact with the gastric juice. The breakdown of starch, catalyzed by salivary amylase, will therefore continue for some time in the stomach. The pH optimum for amylase is 7, but the hydrolysis will continue at a considerable rate until the pH falls to 4·5. This phase of gastric digestion is called the amylotic phase. Carbohydrases of the food will also be active in this period. Through the action of these enzymes starch and other polysaccharides are broken down to di- and monosaccharides. Cellulose is not digested in the stomach.

As the gastric juice penetrates the food the pH falls. This inhibits amylase and stimulates the action of pepsin which has its pH optimum at about 2. During this phase, the amylo-proteolytic phase, both starch and protein, are broken down. When the pH falls further amylase is completely inhibited and only pepsin is active. During this phase, the proteolytic phase, protein is hydrolyzed to polypeptides.

DIGESTION IN THE SMALL INTESTINE

The small intestine is composed of duodenum, jejunum and ileum. By peristaltic movement the food is mixed and moved through the intestinal tract. Two large glands open into the duodenum, the liver and the pancreas.

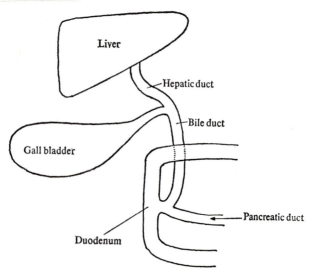

Fig.7.3. The bile system which carries bile from the liver to the duodenum (Horrobin).

There is a continuous secretion of bile by the liver. This bile is stored in the gall bladder (except in horses where the gall bladder is

Table 7.2 Principal enzymes of the digestive tract

Origin	Enzyme	Precursor	Activator	Substrate	End Product
Saliva	Ptyalin (α-amylase)	—	—	Starch,	Dextrins, maltose
Gastric juice	Pepsin (proteases)	Pepsinogen	Hydro-chloric acid	Proteins	Proteoses, peptones
Gastric juice	Rennin	Renninogen (Prorennin)	Hydro-chloric acid	Casein	Calcium caseinate Proteoses, peptones
Pancreatic juice	Trypsin	Trypsinogen	Enterokinase	Proteins, proteoses	Peptones, peptides
Pancreatic juice	Chymo-trypsin	Chymo-trypsinogen	Trypsin	Proteins, proteoses	Peptones, peptides
Pancreatic juice	Carboxy-peptidases	Pro-carboxy-peptidase	Trypsin	Peptides	Amino acids
Pancreatic juice	Amino peptidases	Proamino-peptidase	Trypsin	Peptides	Amino acids
Pancreatic juice	Lipase	—	—	Fats	Glycerides, fatty acids
Pancreatic juice	Maltase	—	—	Maltose	Glucose
Pancreatic juice	Sucrase	—	—	Sucrose	Glucose, fructose
Pancreatic juice	Amylase	—	—	Starch	Dextrins, maltose
Pancreatic juice	Nuclease	—	—	Nucleic acids	Nucleotides
Succus entericus	Amino peptidases	—	—	Proteoses, peptones	Amino acids
Succus entericus	Dipep-tidases	—	—	Proteoses, peptones	Amino acids
Succus entericus	Maltase	—	—	Maltose	Glucose
Succus entericus	Lactase	—	—	Lactose	Glucose
Succus entericus	Sucrase	—	—	Sucrose	Glucose, fructose
Succus entericus	Nuclease	—	—	Nucleic acid	Purine and pyrimidine bases, phosphoric acid, pentose sugars
Succus entericus	Nucleo-tidase	—	—	Nucleic acid	

absent). By an appropriate stimulus the gall bladder contracts and delivers its contents into the duodenum.

Bile is a brownish viscid fluid containing the bile salts and various organic substances. The bile salts are sodium and potassium salts of glycocholic or taurocholic acid. The major organic compounds are phospholipids, cholesterol, and the bile pigments bilirubin and biliverdin. The reaction of the bile is weakly alkaline with a pH between 7 and 8.

Bile salts, together with the lipids of the bile, play an important role in the intestinal digestion of lipids, in that the feed lipids are turned into a coarse stable emulsion. This emulsion is easily attacked by the pancreatic enzymes. Various compounds are capable of stimulating bile formation from the liver. Of major importance is the stimulation by reabsorbed bile salts. Also absorbed fats and amino acids will increase bile formation during the digestive periods. As already mentioned, the presence of food in the duodenum causes release of the hormone secretin. In addition to stimulating gastric secretion, secretin has a marked stimulatory effect on bile formation.

The application of dilute acids or fats to the duodenum causes contraction of the gall bladder and subsequently delivery of bile to

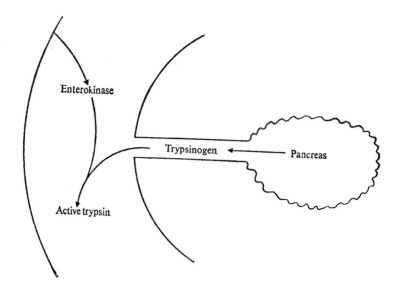

Fig.7.4. The activation of trypsinogen by enterokinase in the intestine (Horrobin).

the intestine. The bladder contraction is due to stimulation by a hormone which is also released from the duodenal mucosa. This hormone is known as cholecystokinin.

The secretion from the pancreas is a clear, distinctly alkaline liquid which contains several proteolytic, and amylolytic enzymes. The alkalinity is due to bicarbonate which is of importance in neutralizing the acid digesta from the stomach.

The proteolytic enzymes of the pancreatic juice include trypsin, chymotrypsin, and carboxypeptidase. Trypsin is secreted as the inactive compound trypsinogen, which is converted into trypsin by calcium ions and enterokinase (Fig.7.4). The conversion of trypsinogen to trypsin is autocatalytic and small amounts of trypsin will catalyze the conversion. Chymotrypsin is also secreted as an inactive zymogen, chymotrypsinogen. The conversion of this compound into chymotrypsin is catalyzed by trypsin. Both trypsin and chymotrypsin are endopeptidases which hydrolyze peptide in the interior of the peptide chain, whereas carboxypeptidases attack the peptide bonds from the carboxyl end of the chain. Like the other two enzymes carboxypeptidase is secreted as a zymogen, a procarboxypeptidase.

Pancreatic lipase acts specifically to remove the fatty acid residues linked to alpha-hydroxyl groups of glycerol. The action of this enzyme thus causes the formation of beta-monoglycerides and free fatty acids.

Pancreatic amylase can convert starch to the disaccharide maltose. The maltose is further broken down to glucose by the enzyme maltase, also secreted from the pancreas.

The secretion of pancreatic juice is under the influence of two hormones produced by the mucosa of the duodenum in response to stimulation by chyme (Fig.7.5). The hormone secretin increases the rate of flow and the bicarbonate concentration in the pancreatic juice in response to acid from the stomach. Pancreozymin increases the amount of enzymes in the pancreatic juice in response to lipids in the duodenum. Stimulation of the vagal nerve will also cause the pancreas to secrete a juice rich in enzymes, similar to that produced by pancreozymin. This neural control is reflexly stimulated by eating. All pancreatic enzymes have their pH optimum at 8 (Table 7.1).

The secretion from the intestinal glands (Brunner's glands in the duodenum and the crypts of Lieberkuhn in the jejunum) appears to be a continuous process although it increases following a meal. In

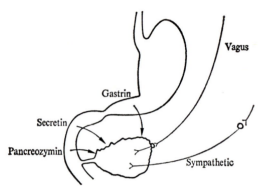

Fig.7.5. The control of pancreatic secretion (from Horrobin, *Medical Physiology and Biochemistry*, by kind permission of the author and Edward Arnold, 1968).

pigs this increase follows a flat curve with its maximum 1–2 hours after feeding and the minimum 8 hours later. The intestinal secretion is stimulated by two hormones released from the mucosa of the duodenum, secretin and enterocrinin.

The pH of the intestinal secretion ranges from 7·4–8·7. It contains several enzymes: enterokinase, which activates trypsinogen to trypsin, maltase, which hydrolyzes maltose to glucose, sucrase, which hydrolyzes sucrose to glucose and fructose, lactase, which hydrolyzes lactose to glucose and galactose, peptidases, which hydrolyze peptides to amino acids, and several others which reduce the size of the organic molecules in the intestinal contents.

As a result of the combined enzymatic digestion the proteins are broken down to amino acids, the lipids to a mixture of free fatty acids, beta-monoglycerides, and small amounts of alpha-diglycerides and triglycerides, and the digestible carbohydrates are broken down primarily to glucose, and to a smaller extent to fructose, galactose, and other monosaccharides.

DIGESTION IN THE LARGE INTESTINE

In omnivorous and herbivorous animals the caecum and colon are relatively large organs, whereas in carnivorous animals they are of smaller size. The secretion from the crypts of Lieberkuhn in the mucosa of the large intestine is not very copious; it has a high mucin content but contains no significant amounts of digestive enzymes. In pigs and especially horses the intestinal digestion is continued in the large intestine by the action of bacterial enzymes. This bacterial fermentation in the intestinal tract leads to formation of substances which are waste products for the bacteria but of value to the host animal. In this way the simple stomached animals are capable of utilizing, to some extent, the cellulose ingested. The products of the bacterial fermentation of cellulose are the volatile fatty acids, namely acetic, propionic, and butyric acid. Detailed information on the processes leading to the formation of the volatile fatty acids will be given in the chapter on ruminant digestion.

The nutritional value of feeding cellulose to pigs is rather small if at all significant. Of much greater importance to the animal is the bacterial synthesis of dietary essentials, especially B-vitamins.

It is evident that the addition of antibiotics to the ration may have considerable influence upon the microbial activity in the gastro-intestinal tract. The beneficial effect which is sometimes observed by the addition may be due especially to a depression of pathological micro-organisms. The advantage of a general and continuous addition of antibiotics to swine rations is, for many reasons, doubtful.

The rate of passage through the gastro-intestinal tract varies with the composition of the ration. Since fats delay gastric emptying, rations rich in lipids pass more slowly through the tract than do lipid poor rations. When pigs are given a test meal containing a coloured compound, the excretion of the compound will begin about 12 hours after the meal and about 60 per cent will be excreted by the end of the second 12 hour period. Three to four days are required for complete excretion.

When the contents in the ampulla of the rectum have accumulated to a certain extent, the defecation reflex is initiated. This reflex involves involuntary as well as voluntary muscles. When the sphincter muscles of the anus are relaxed the emptying of the rectum is accomplished by tonic contraction of muscles in the rectal wall and by contraction of the abdominal muscles.

The faeces are composed of water, indigestible food residues, remains of digestive secretions, desquamated epithelial cells, and numerous bacteria. The composition and amount of faeces vary with the feed ingested.

8

Digestion in ruminants

In the animal kingdom there is a remarkable lack of ability to degrade cellulose enzymatically. This is an extraordinary feature of animal evolution as so many animals are herbivorous in their feeding habits. In those species capable of using cellulose as an important source of energy, some modification of the gastro-intestinal tract is found to harbour symbiotic micro-organisms that can break down cellulose to compounds useful to the host animal. In horses and similar herbivorous animals the caecum and part of the colon have developed into large hollow organs suitable for bacterial growth. The results of the microbial processes, however, cannot be utilized to their full extent. The fermentation products—the volatile fatty acids—may to some extent be absorbed, but the micro-organisms themselves and with them a valuable source of protein are lost in the faeces.

In ruminants the gastro-intestinal tract is well adapted for micro-bial fermentation and utilization of the end products of this ferment-ation. The stomach has evolved into a complex of four chambers. The true stomach, or the abomasum, is similar to the stomach of simple stomached animals. It consists of the usual fundic and pyloric regions, with typical glands producing digestive enzymes and hydrochloric acid. The area of the secretory mucosa is enlarged by a number of soft folds extending into the lumen.

The cardiac region has become modified into three compartments, rumen, reticulum, and omasum. The rumen and the reticulum form a single functional unit, though the form of the two compartments and the appearance of the mucous membrane make anatomical differentiation quite easy. From the cardia of the rumen a well defined muscular groove, the reticular groove, passes down the medial wall of the reticulum to the reticulo-omasal orifice. In the young ruminant the lips of the reticular groove close to form a tube during suckling to ensure that milk passes directly from the oesophagus, via the reticular groove and the omasal canal, to the abomasum. In the adult ruminant the reticular groove does not play any essential role. The omasum is the most modified of the compartments. At the base of the organ, a narrow canal passes from the reticulo-omasal orifice to the omaso–abomasal orifice. The opening and closure of these two openings is controlled by the relative position of the three stomach compartments. The remaining part of the omasum, the omasal body, is a firm ball-shaped structure. The inner surface is very large, as there are numerous leaves extending from the dorsal wall towards the omasal canal.

The small intestine and the digestive glands are similar to those of the non-ruminants. The large intestine in general resembles that of the omnivore, having a rather large caecum and a long but simple colon, which is coiled into a double spiral.

PREHENSION AND MASTICATION

The ruminants have developed a unique dental apparatus for prehension of their plant food. The maxillary incisors are lacking and are replaced by a hard pad on which the mandibular incisors can bite. A distinct interdermal space separates the incisors from the molars which are well adapted for the grinding necessary to comminute coarse plant fragments. The secretion of saliva in ruminants is so great that the animal does not need to drink water while eating even the driest food. The daily secretion in cattle is between 40 and 60 litres. The saliva contains no enzymes, but large amounts of phosphorus and bicarbonate which provide the principal fluid medium for microbial growth and fermentation. Phosphorus is present chiefly in inorganic form and has a concentration that may exceed ten times that in the blood. The high phosphorus concentration is favourable to bacterial growth as well as important as a buffer in the rumen fluid. The bicarbonate of the saliva acts as the principal buffer in the rumen fluid, neutralizing the fermentation acids and thus maintaining the ruminal pH near 6.

During grazing, the ruminant collects the food quite rapidly, chews only sufficiently to prepare a suitable bolus, and then swallows. In rest periods the digesta from the rumen is regurgitated and re-chewed to facilitate bacterial action.

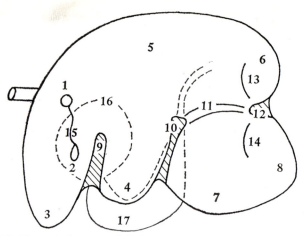

Fig.8.1. The reticulo-rumen, left view. (1) Cardia. (2) Reticulo-omasal orifice. (3) Reticulum. (4) Cranial sac of rumen. (5) Dorsal sac of rumen. (6) Caudodorsal blindsac. (7) Ventral sac of rumen. (8) Ventral caudal blindsac. (9) Rumino-reticular fold. (10) Cranial pillar. (11) Right longitudinal pillar. (12) Caudal pillar. (13) Dorsal coronary pillar. (14) Ventral coronary pillar. (15) Reticular groove. (16) Omasum (on opposite side). (17) Abomasum.

GASTRIC MOVEMENTS IN THE RUMINANT

Mixing of the rumen-reticular contents aids in inoculating fresh ingesta with the mass of micro-organisms in the fermenting digesta. It helps to spread saliva throughout the rumen, it enhances absorption by replenishing the fermentation acids already absorbed by the rumen epithelium, and it assists the passage of digesta to other organs of the alimentary tract. The mixing is accomplished by contractions of the walls of the rumen and reticulum, coordinated with movements of other digestive organs.

The basic or primary mixing cycle consists of a fairly regular sequence of events occurring about once every minute, more often in small ruminants, and at an increased rate during feeding or rumination.

The cycle starts with two successive contractions of the reticulum (3) (Fig.8.1). The first of these lasts 2–3 seconds. The second, which is complete, occurs before the reticulum has entirely relaxed from the first contraction. After the second contraction, the reticulum relaxes. At the time of the first reticular contraction the rumino-reticular fold (9) contracts, and with the second contraction both the fold (9), the cranial pillar (10), and the caudal pillar (12) contract.

When the reticulum relaxes after its second contraction, the wall of the dorsal sac of the rumen (5) contracts. Cranial and caudal pillars (10, 12) are fully contracted, as are the dorsal coronary pillar (13), the longitudinal pillar (11), and the caudodorsal blindsac (6). The ventral coronary pillar (14) and the ventral sac of the rumen (7) are relaxed. During this stage digesta will be forced from the dorsal to the ventral part of the rumen.

The last contractions of the mixing cycle occur in the ventral sac (7), the ventral coronary pillar (14), and the caudoventral blindsac (8). This series of events causes the liquid in the ventral portion to rise around the main mass of digesta, percolate into it, and mix with the more solid materials. The rising liquid also spills over into the reticulum and carries with it some of the smaller solids. As a result of these mixing movements the reticulum usually contains more liquid and less solid material than does the rumen, and the particles tend to be finer. The coarse particles of the digesta will remain in the cranial end of the dorsal sac.

In addition to the sequence of muscular movements described above, there are often intercalated one or more rumen contractions in addition to those directly following the two reticular contraction. These are known as secondary contractions and related to the eructation of rumen gas.

Rumination

The process of rechewing the food or chewing the cud is one of the most distinctive features of the ruminants. It is intimately connected with the use of herbage as food.

As the first step in rumination, digesta in the rumen is regurgitated into the mouth. Regurgitation is initiated by contact of coarse particles with the area around the opening of the oesophagus into the rumen, and accomplished by a complicated set of muscular contractions preceding the two reticular contractions of a mixing cycle. The cardia (1) (Fig.8.1) opens and the animal inspires against a closed glottis. This creates a lower than atmospheric pressure in the pleural cavity and since the oesophagus is quite pliable the decreased pressure is transmitted to the interior of the oesophagus. As a result of the pressure difference between the rumen and the oesophagus, digesta enters the oesophagus. The cardia closes and the bolus is brought to the mouth by reverse peristalsis. The liquid accompanying the solids is immediately swallowed in one or two portions, and the solids are chewed. The rechewing during rumination is more thorough than the initial mastication during feeding. The jaws operate with a lateral grinding motion, and each bolus is chewed from 30–85 times depending on the nature of the feed. The total time of chewing one bolus varies from 25–60 seconds. During rumination there is an increase in secretion of saliva.

The rechewed bolus is swallowed and another regurgitated almost immediately. Since each regurgitation precedes the initiation of the primary cycle, rumination is synchronized with the contraction cycle in that one bolus is rechewed per cycle. The swallowed ruminated bolus enters and mixes in the rumen in the same fashion as boluses swallowed during feeding. There are no means for shunting the rechewed digesta directly to the omasum. Since there is no complete separation of ruminated from unruminated digesta, some material may enter more than one rumination cycle.

Direct observations on grazing cattle have shown that the maximum time spent on rumination is about 8 hours per 24 hours. Each bolus contains about 100 g of material, which means that about 50 kg of digesta are rechewed each day.

The result of rumination is a reduction in particle size of the food to facilitate passage through the alimentary tract, and to permit the complete action of the microbial digestive enzymes.

Eructation

Methane and carbon dioxide are metabolic products of the rumen fermentation, and carbon dioxide is also liberated from bicarbonate by acidification. This copious production of gas (approximately 800 litres of CO_2 and 500 litres of CH_4 each 24 hours in a cow, necessitates a mechanism for its escape. About a quarter of the gas escapes via the blood and lungs to the expired air. The remaining part is voided by eructation.

The secondary rumen contractions have been mentioned previously. Each of these additional contractions immediately precedes an eructation. The secondary contraction is chiefly in the dorsal sac, and it causes the large gas volume above the rumen digesta to be displaced forward. At the same time the rumino-reticular fold contracts and holds back the forward surge of solid digesta. These movements cause the gas to move into the dorsal part of the reticulum. The cardia then opens, and the gas escapes through the oesophagus (Fig.8.3).

Separation of coarse from fine particles

The material leaving the rumen is not representative of the total
rumen contents. Comparison of the size of particles in rumen digesta
with those in the faeces of hay fed animals shows only fine particles
in the latter, as compared to the many large plant fragments in the
rumen. There is a mechanism for partial retention of coarse particles
in the rumen and a very effective mechanism for their complete
retention in the reticulum.

The partial separation of coarse from fine particles between the
rumen and the reticulum is caused in part by the rapid reticular
contractions that expel into the rumen the coarse material which
floats on top, in part by the contraction of the ventral sac of the
rumen by which liquid wells up and around the mass of solid digesta
and spills over into the reticulum.

The reticulo-omasal orifice is the site of complete separation of
coarse from fine particles. The fine ones pass into the omasum, the
coarse ones accumulate due to the screening action of the orifice,
and lie in a favourable position for regurgitation. They will have
accumulated to a maximum just before the next mixing cycle starts,
which is also the time when rumination occurs.

Reticular groove

In the newborn ruminant the abomasum is relatively larger than the
other compartments. It receives milk directly from the oesophagus
via the reticular groove and the omasal canal, which function as a
bypass of the rumen–reticulum. The act of suckling induces reflex
contractions of the muscles in the ridges extending along each side
of the reticular groove and in the groove itself. These contractions
narrow the gap between the two longitudinal ridges and shorten the
groove with a twisting motion which closes the gap to form a tube
joining the oesophagus with the omasum.

If the young animal drinks milk from a bucket, the amount
swallowed at one time may force open the closed reticular groove
and allow milk to enter the rumen. Here it undergoes a lactic acid
fermentation and gives an acid reaction to the rumen contents,
which may cause diarrhoea. This can be avoided by feeding smaller
amounts several times daily.

MOVEMENTS OF THE OMASUM

The omasum acts as a one-way pump that allows digesta to pass
from the reticulum to the abomasum. At the height of the second

4

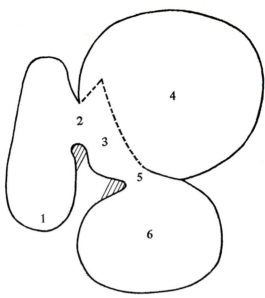

Fig.8.2. Transection of the ruminant stomach viewed from behind. (1) Reticulum. (2) Reticulo-omasal orifice. (3) Omasal canal. (4) Omasal body. (5) Omasoabomasal orifice. (6) Abomasum.

reticular (Fig.8.2,1) contraction in the primary mixing cycle the reticulo-omasal orifice (2) opens and a gush of digesta passes into the omasal canal (3). The orifice then closes and a strong contraction of the canal forces digesta into the body of the omasum (4) between the leaves. This occurs simultaneously with the contraction of the dorsal sac of the rumen. The omasal body is filled after several canal contractions. At irregular intervals the omasoabomasal orifice (5) opens and the omasal body contracts, expelling the contents into the abomasum.

THE ABOMASUM

Functionally the abomasum differs greatly from the stomach of simple stomached animals. The material that reaches the abomasum has been extensively digested in the forestomach. It contains only small particles and is received in small quantities throughout the entire day. Although volume changes occur according to the digestability of the feed, the abomasal volume and flow rate are maintained at fairly steady levels and the organ is never emptied under ordinary feeding conditions.

In accordance with the continuous passage through the abomasum, there is a continuous secretion of gastric juice. This secretion is not stimulated by feeding, the principal stimulus is provided by the flow of digesta from the omasum, and the release of gastrin from the mucous membrane of the pyloric part. The principal factor affecting the release of gastrin is the pH of the abomasal digesta. The digesta coming from the omasum is only slightly acid and highly buffered, and tends to raise the pH of the abomasal contents. This stimulates the release of gastrin and thus the secretion of hydrochloric acid. A low pH inhibits the release of gastrin, and acid secretion declines. This inhibition occurs when the pH reaches 2. This mechanism tends to maintain the abomasal reaction rather constant at a pH near 2·5. The rate of flow of digesta into the abomasum is controlled

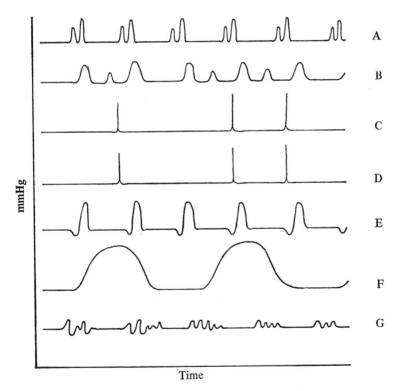

Fig.8.3. Pressure recordings from the ruminant stomach. (A) Reticulum. (B) Rumen. (C) Thoracic oesophagus. (D) Cervical oesophagus. (E) Omasal canal. (F) Omasal body. (G) Abomasum.

by parasympathetic reflexes. Increased rumen volume causes an increased flow rate, whereas distension of the abomasum inhibits the flow of digesta. Similarly, distension and emptying of the duodenum controls the flow rate through the pylorus.

The high acidity of the abomasal juice causes instant destruction of the micro-organisms that reach the abomasum from the rumen, allowing the proteolytic enzymes to attack the microbial protein to yield amino acids. This probably constitutes the main function of the abomasum.

THE INTESTINES

The characteristic feature of the ruminant small intestine is its length. Functionally there is no important difference from the simple stomached animals. The large intestine resembles that of omnivorous animals. Caecum and colon serve as a fermentation chamber with a high bacterial activity. Cellulose and other carbohydrates that have escaped fermentation in the rumen may be broken down in the large intestine, and the fermentation products utilized by the animal.

MICROBIAL DIGESTION IN THE RUMEN

In the simple stomached animal the digestive enzymes merely break down the complex structures of the feed into smaller units that can be absorbed and metabolized. In ruminants, the feed taken is primarily utilized by the vast number of micro-organisms in the rumen. The waste products of this microbial digestion, the volatile fatty acids, are absorbed by the host and serve as a source of energy. The micro-organisms themselves are carried to the abomasum, where they are denatured by the acid. The microbial protein is hydrolyzed by proteolytic enzymes, and the resulting amino acids are absorbed by the ruminant. The loss of energy in this process is considerable, the gains being that the ruminants can derive energy from cellulose, and that they can resynthesize high quality protein from protein of lower biological value. This makes ruminants less dependent on the amino acid composition in their feed than simple stomached animals.

Rumen bacteria

The rumen bacteria are adapted to live at acidities between pH 5·5 and 7·0, in the absence of oxygen, at a temperature of 39–40 °C, in the presence of moderate concentrations of fermentation products, and at the expense of the ingesta provided by the ruminant. The steady supply of food and continuous removal of fermentation products and food residues maintain relatively constant conditions in which an extremely dense population of bacteria lives, a population in the order of 10^{10} per g rumen contents.

The rumen bacteria ferment carbohydrate and protein from the feed. The fermentation consists in rearrangement of the atoms into molecules in which some carbon atoms are more oxidized and others are more reduced.

Cellulose and hemicellulose digesting bacteria

Cellulose digesting bacteria break down cellulose mainly to acetic acid, lactic acid, butyric acid, and smaller amounts of propionic acid. The cellulolytic bacteria apply themselves to the fibres of the plant material and secrete a depolymerizing enzyme. This results in the formation of microscopic pockets in which the bacteria are found. The very close proximity of the bacteria to the point at which soluble products are released, enables them to absorb the breakdown products before they diffuse away into the surrounding medium. The digestion of cellulose is a rather slow process, and the concentration of bacteria in the rumen fluid and that of fermentation products increases only slightly, if at all, following a meal rich in cellulose. This indicates that the formation of bacteria and production of fermentation acids equals absorption and outflow.

Hemicellulose is a plant carbohydrate that constitutes a large percentage of the feed consumed by ruminants. It undergoes digestion in the rumen to about the same extent as cellulose. The fermentation products are acetic acid, butyric acid, and smaller amounts of propionic acid.

Starch digesting bacteria

A number of microbial enzymes, capable of completely degrading starch, are produced by rumen microbes. Microscopic examination shows that bacteria apply themselves to starch granules and steadily erode the structure. The products of starch fermentation are propionic acid, lactic acid, and smaller amounts of acetic and butyric acids. Animals on high grain rations develop very high concentrations of starch digesting bacteria in the rumen fluid. This increases the fermentation rate and the concentration of the fermentation products increases, indicating that the production exceeds the absorption and outflow. If an animal overeats grain, the concentration of lactic acid will build up in the rumen causing severe sickness, known as grain overload or rumen acidosis.

Under normal conditions only trace amounts of lactic acid are present in the rumen although it is produced in large quantities by several organisms. The reason for this is that lactic acid is a nutrient for several rumen bacteria and yields the usual volatile fatty acids. Lactic acid is thus a major precursor in the formation of propionic acid.

Soluble sugar digesting bacteria

All of the polysaccharide digesting bacteria can also utilize mono- or disaccharides. The fermentation products are acetic, lactic, and butyric acids.

Protein digesting bacteria

Proteolytic bacteria break down proteins and amino acids to yield volatile fatty acids and ammonia. The ammonia in turn is utilized for synthesis of microbial protein.

Rumen protozoa

Besides the bacteria in the rumen, a large number of single celled organisms, protozoa, are found. Most of these are ciliates, but a few species of small flagellates are also found. The rumen protozoa have evolved into a highly specialized group fitted to survive only in the rumen. They are anaerobic, can ferment constituents of plant materials for energy, and can grow at rumen temperatures in the presence of billions of accompanying bacteria.

The protozoa utilize mainly starch, and form acetic, propionic, butyric, and lactic acids as the chief fermentation acids. The proportion of these acids varies in the different species.

CARBOHYDRATE FERMENTATION

The carbohydrates eaten by the ruminant are digested by the rumen micro-organisms to supply energy for their growth and reproduction. The waste products of this digestion are the volatile fatty acids (VFA), CO_2, and CH_4. Although the rumen VFA are waste products and of no value for the micro-organisms, they can be utilized by the host.

The result of carbohydrate fermentation is a rise in the number of rumen micro-organisms and a rise in the concentration of VFA. The relative concentration of the three acids depends both on the composition of the feed and on the physical form of the feed. A diet rich in cellulose will yield a relatively larger amount of acetic acid, whereas a starch rich ration will yield more propionic acid and suppress the formation of acetic acid. If ruminants are given all their roughage in a finely ground form, the production of acetic acid falls and the production of propionic acid rises, compared to feeding the same ration unground. The acetate : propionate ratio in the rumen is of importance, mainly because acetate after absorption enters the lipid metabolism as a precursor in the synthesis of milk fat, whereas propionate enters into the carbohydrate metabolism as the primary supplier of energy.

The rumen VFA concentration varies between 60 and 120 mEq per 1, and the average molar percentage of the acids are: acetic 62, propionic 22, and butyric 16.

The overall result of the carbohydrate fermentation in the rumen is that practically all soluble carbohydrates and the major part (60–90 per cent) of the starch are broken down to volatile fatty acids. The amount of cellulose digested depends on the composition of the feed. If it contains large amounts of easily digestible carbohydrates, the digestion of cellulose will be depressed. Small amounts of starch, however, increase the utilization of cellulose. Under normal feeding conditions approximately 50–60 per cent of the ingested cellulose, hemicellulose, and pectin will be digested in the rumen. The remaining part will undergo microbial fermentation in the caecum and colon, or appear in the faeces.

As the carbohydrate fermentation in the rumen is a result of microbial action, any condition that increases the number of micro-organisms will increase the rate of digestion. It is therefore essential that the feed contains the necessary nitrogen containing substances to ensure synthesis of bacterial protein.

CONVERSION OF NITROGENOUS MATERIALS

The nitrogen containing substances in the feed are composed of proteins, amino acids, and lower organic and inorganic compounds.

Protein and amino acids

Proteins are the most common nitrogenous material in forages. The first step in protein utilization is digestion. In theory, it would seem

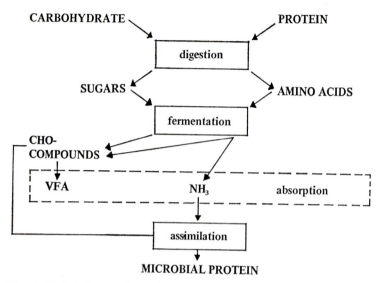

Fig.8.4. Carbohydrate and protein interrelationship in the rumen.

simplest and most profitable for the rumen micro-organisms to digest the food proteins and assimilate the amino acids directly into microbial protein, using the high energy phosphate available from fermentation. The amino acids of the food protein would then become the amino acids of the microbe. This occurs to some degree, but proteins are mainly used in other ways. Some rumen bacteria use the amino acids of protein to yield high energy phosphate. The nitrogen is removed, and the carbon and hydrogen containing residues are rearranged in much the same fashion as that in which carbohydrates are fermented. When amino acids are fermented to provide energy, ammonia is formed. The ammonia may in turn again be assimilated into amino acids if carbohydrate is available. The relative importance of proteins for cell synthesis depends on the ratio of carbohydrate to nitrogen in the rumen (Fig.8.4).

The degree to which protein is digested in the rumen depends on the solubility of the protein in the rumen fluid. Soluble proteins are more readily attacked than insoluble proteins. This is of importance as the insoluble proteins have a greater opportunity of leaving the rumen without being degraded and resynthesized into microbial protein. This will influence the biological value of the feed protein, depending on whether it has a higher or lower value than the microbial protein. Normally between 40 and 50 per cent of the ingested protein undergoes proteolytic digestion in the rumen. The remaining part undergoes enzymatic digestion in the abomasum and intestine.

Ammonia

The foregoing account of the fermentation of amino acids indicates that ammonia is always formed during the process. One of the most intriguing problems in rumen physiology is the extent to which ammonia serves as the nitrogenous material for synthesis of microbial protein. Many signs point in the direction of importance: (1) ammonia appears rapidly in the rumen contents when the feed contains much nitrogen. (2) many rumen bacteria assimilate NH_3 in preference to amino acids. (3) considerable quantities of feed ammonia can be assimilated by the host animal, presumably via assimilation by the rumen microbes. (4) tracer studies with ^{15}N have shown incorporation of ammonia into amino acids by rumen bacteria.

This indicates a capacity for ammonia utilization by rumen micro-organisms. The next question is the extent to which this capacity is utilized. When ruminants are fed starch and soluble sugars, both soluble proteins and soluble carbohydrates will be present in the rumen shortly after the meal is ingested. Digestion of the protein is rapid, with release of amino acids which may be assimilated directly. When a feed rich in fibre is ingested the bacteria grow more slowly and during the extended period in which they attack the more resistant components, the proteins are broken down to amino acids and further to ammonia. It is thus not surprising that the fibre digesting bacteria have a well developed ability to assimilate ammonia into microbial protein.

Urea

As in all other mammals, the saliva of ruminants contains urea at a concentration of about 70 per cent of that in the blood. The very large volume of saliva in ruminants makes this addition of urea to the rumen of great significance. Further, urea tends to diffuse across the rumen wall from the blood to the lumen, and in this way an even larger volume reaches the rumen digesta. Urea is thus normally ingested and enters the rumen continuously. It is therefore not surprising to find the enzyme urease in the rumen. This enzyme, produced by the micro-organisms, converts urea to carbon dioxide and ammonia. Part of the ammonia is assimilated into microbial protein while the rest is absorbed and converted into urea by the liver. Part of this urea is excreted by the kidneys, and part of it reaches the rumen again. This chain of reactions is known as the urea-ammonia cycle.

The degree to which urea can supplement protein in the ruminant diet depends on the amount of carbohydrate available and the amount of other nitrogen sources in the feed. If the ruminant receives a ration containing all necessities except protein, and with plenty of digestible carbohydrate, there is a net assimilation of nitrogen from urea. In practice, it is usually found that urea can supply about one third of the required nitrogen. Instances in which urea supplementation does not significantly improve growth, may be due to a lack of carbohydrate, minerals, or an excess of other nitrogen sources.

LIPIDS

In the ruminal digestion of lipids, special interest attaches to the hydrogenation of unsaturated fatty acids. Hydrolysis of esterified fatty acids also occurs, and the free glycerol formed is readily fermented. The mechanism of this hydrogenation is not fully known. It is, however, believed that the hydrogen released by the fermentation of carbohydrates and proteins is activated by a microbial hydrogenase.

The micro-organisms leaving the rumen contribute to the animal's intake of lipid as some 9 per cent of the dry weight of the rumen bacteria is lipid.

RESULTS OF RUMEN DIGESTION

The reactions of the rumen microbes reduce the complex mixture of the feed to a number of smaller molecules, that can readily be absorbed and metabolized by the ruminant. While in the simple stomached animal the feed is broken down to monosaccharides, amino acids, and fatty acids, in the ruminant the end products of digestion are acetic, propionic, and butyric acids, long chain fatty acids, ammonia, and the gases carbon dioxide and methane. These few substances, together with the bodies of the micro-organisms themselves, comprise the bulk of the ruminant's real food.

Fats are only found in small amounts in most ruminant feeds and hence the long chain fatty acids of the ruminal digesta make only a small contribution to the animal's nutrition. The ammonia that does not assimilate into protein is absorbed and excreted or recycled, and

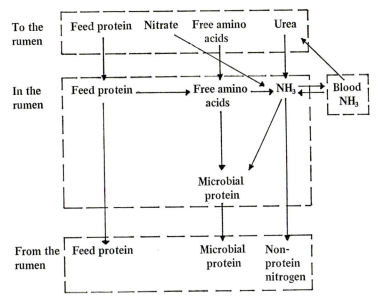

Fig.8.5. The digestion of nitrogenous substances in the rumen.

carbon dioxide and methane are lost by eructation. The three volatile fatty acids are left to make the chief contribution to the ruminant's energy intake. The micro-organisms are denatured by the acid in the abomasum, and serve as the chief source of protein to the animal.

The food that escapes microbial digestion in the rumen will either be broken down by enzymes in the abomasum and small intestine (protein, starch, and soluble sugar), or it will undergo microbial fermentation in the cecum and colon. Under normal feeding conditions very little of the feed ingested reaches the abomasum without being completely fermented by the rumen micro-organisms, except for cellulose of which about 20 per cent is digested in the caecum.

9

Absorption and metabolism

ABSORPTION FROM THE GASTRO-INTESTINAL TRACT

Digestion and gastro-intestinal movements prepare the food for absorption through the epithelium of the digestive canal. Absorption might thus be considered the central function of the intestinal canal. Absorption mainly takes place from the small intestine, except in ruminants where the forestomach is an important site of absorption.

A number of general considerations govern absorption across any surface: (1) the transport may be active or passive. Passive transport or diffusion is said to take place when substances flow from a region of high concentration to a region of low concentration, or if the substance is electrically charged and the particles move toward charge of opposite sign. Transport against the electrochemical gradient requires energy, and is defined as active transport; (2) the amount of material transported across the epithelium depends on the surface area involved. The gastro-intestinal surface area is increased by large mucosal folds, by small projections known as villi, and by microvilli which project from the surface of the epithelial cells; (3) the size of the electrochemical gradient will determine the rate of passive as well as of active transport. Active forces can only move material if the opposing gradient is not too great. If it is too great, the passive movement down the gradient will exceed the active movement against the gradient. (4) the intestinal lumen is about 3–10 mV and the rumen lumen about 16 mV negative to the blood, mainly because of the rapid active transport of the positively charged sodium ions; (5) absorption will occur only if the epithelium is permeable to the material concerned; in general the greater the particle size, the less the membrane permeability. Lipid solubility increases permeability.

Absorption of sodium (Na$^+$)

The rumen and intestinal walls are highly permeable to sodium and there are large passive movements in both directions. The electrochemical gradient will determine whether the net movement is into or out of the digestive tract. Superimposed upon these passive movements is an active mechanism by which sodium can move against the electrochemical gradient from mucosal side to serosal side. The active process, however, cannot remove all the sodium from the lumen. The epithelium is so permeable that when the luminal sodium concentration is low, the passive flux into the lumen is equal to the sum of the active and passive flux out of the lumen. The limiting luminal concentration is about 65 mEq/1. At luminal concentrations above this sodium is absorbed, at concentrations below this level, it passes from the blood to the lumen (Fig.9.1).

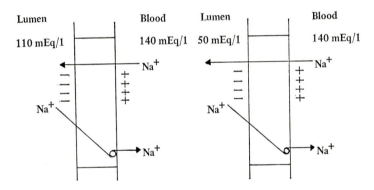

Fig.9.1. Absorption and loss of sodium in the gastro-intestinal tract (see text).

Absorption of potassium (K$^+$)

The transport of potassium across the gastro-intestinal epithelium is a passive process down the concentration gradient but against the electrical gradient. Because of the large concentration gradient the net movement will be from the lumen to the blood (Fig.9.2).

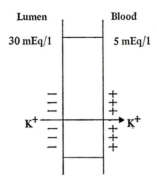

Fig.9.2. Absorption of potassium across the gastro-intestinal tract (see text).

Absorption of chloride (Cl⁻)

The chloride transport is a passive process down the electrical gradient, but against the concentration gradient if the lumen concentration of chloride is above 35 mEq/1. At concentrations below 35 mEq/1 chloride will move the opposite way because the force of the concentration gradient exceeds the force of the electrical gradient (Fig.9.3).

Absorption of sugars

Glucose and galactose are actively transported from the intestinal lumen to the blood. Other sugars are passively absorbed. Fig.9.4 shows the general scheme for the active transport of nutrients. The

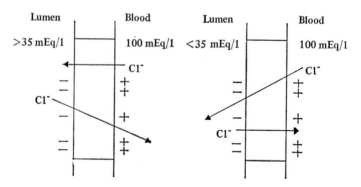

Fig.9.3. Absorption and loss of chloride from the gastro-intestinal tract (see text).

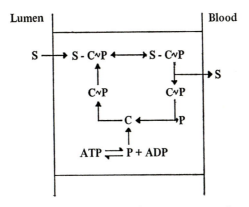

Fig.9.4. Model of 'mobile carrier' membrane transport of nutrients. S = nutrient, C = "mobile carrier", P = H_3PO_4 (see text).

nutrient is bound to a mobile carrier which brings it across the cell membrane into the cytoplasm. The energy required for the formation of the linkage between carrier and nutrient is supplied by hydrolysis of ATP.

Absorption of amino acids

In the newborn mammal the intestinal epithelium is permeable to intact protein molecules, and antibodies ingested with colostrum may thus pass into the blood stream. The blood of the newborn foal, calf, and pig contains almost no gamma-globulin and an early supply of antibodies is therefore of major importance. Within a few days after birth the intestinal epithelium becomes impermeable to protein.

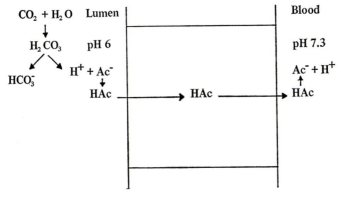

Fig.9.5. Absorption of volatile fatty acids across the rumen epithelium (see text).

This protects the animal against antigens, proteins causing the formation of antibodies and thus allergy and anaphylactic reactions.

Amino acids are absorbed by active transport. Three different 'carriers' have been demonstrated, one for neutral, one for alkaline, and one for acid amino acids. These carrier systems favour the absorption of L-amino acids. From the intestinal epithelium the amino acids are transferred to the liver where they are metabolized.

Absorption of volatile fatty acids

In ruminants the volatile fatty acids are mainly absorbed from the forestomach and the caecum. The undissociated molecules are absorbed much faster than the ionized forms, and thus the rate of absorption increases as the pH is reduced (Fig.9.5). This absorption mechanism tends to maintain the rumen pH at 6. At this pH, the ratio of dissociated to undissociated acid is about 200 : 1, and yet the two forms are absorbed at equal rates. With the absorption of each undissociated molecule of volatile fatty acid, one molecule of bicarbonate appears in the rumen. This leads to a concentration of bicarbonate in the rumen fluid and represents a major mechanism of neutralization of ruminal volatile fatty acids.

Most of the volatile fatty acids produced in the rumen are absorbed in the forestomach and only a minor part passes on to the abomasum. The concentration of volatile fatty acids in the abomasal contents is approximately 10 per cent of that in the rumen.

Absorption of lipids

Most of the lipids are absorbed as free fatty acids and monoglycerides. The longer chain fatty acids (12 or more carbon acids) are absorbed into the lymph. During transport across the epithelium these acids are combined with glycerol to form triglycerides which are then found in the lymph. The shorter chain fatty acids are absorbed into the blood as free fatty acids.

Absorption of water

There are two ways by which water can be moved passively, by difference in hydrostatic pressure between the intestinal lumen and the blood, and by osmotic force. The latter is by far the most important. When sodium ions are actively absorbed from the intestines the number of osmotically active particles in the lumen is reduced. This leaves the intestinal lumen hypotonic to the blood, and so water follows the particles out of the lumen in order to maintain osmotic balance.

METABOLISM

A stack of hay may burn in a matter of hours, with complete waste of the energy. If the same hay is fed to animals, the stepwise controlled oxidation (metabolism) provides enough energy to keep the animals alive and maintain production.

The process which results in building and maintaining body tissue and storage of energy is classified as anabolism. The breakdown of substances, with concurrent release of energy, is known as catabolism.

All energy available to the animals ultimately comes from the sun. Plants utilize this energy in photosynthesis to combine carbon dioxide and water in the formation of plant tissue and consequent storage of energy. The animals obtain this energy directly if they are herbivorous, or indirectly if they are carnivorous. Catabolism of the three major classes of food provides the energy for all vital processes in the animal body. This energy is temporarily stored in the form of so-called 'high energy bonds', which link phosphorus and oxygen atoms in adenosine triphosphate (ATP). In the presence of the appropriate enzymes one phosphate radical splits off, with the release of a great deal of energy. The resulting compound, adenosine diphosphate (ADP), can be converted to ATP by the addition of phosphate and energy

$$ATP + H_2O \rightleftharpoons ADP + H_3PO_4 + ENERGY$$

Metabolism of protein and amino acids

The proteins in the body are in a state of dynamic equilibrium. There is a continuous breakdown and resynthesis of proteins, a catabolism and an anabolism. The amino acids formed by endogenous protein breakdown are in no way different from amino acids derived from digested protein. In the adult, non-pregnant, and non-lactating animal, protein catabolism equals protein anabolism, and the animal is said to be in nitrogen balance. This means that: nitrogen in feed − nitrogen excreted = zero. In a growing animal anabolism normally exceeds catabolism, the animal is in a positive nitrogen balance. If the animal is starved over a prolonged period it will have a negative nitrogen balance.

The amino acids necessary for protein synthesis in the cells are taken from the pool of free amino acids in the blood plasma. This pool is supported by the amino acids absorbed by the intestine, amino acids derived from the breakdown of tissue protein, and amino acids synthesized in the liver. The concentration of amino acids in the plasma varies between 45 and 60 mg per 100 ml.

The synthesis of protein is a complicated process in which amino acids are linked together in a constant sequence depending on the specific protein. The synthesis takes place in the cytoplasm of the cells on the surface of the ribosomes, where the sequence is coded by the bases of ribonucleic acid. The protein synthesis is greater in young animals than in adults on the same diet. This demonstrates that protein synthesis is to some extent independent of the ingested protein, and is a function of the physiological state of the animal.

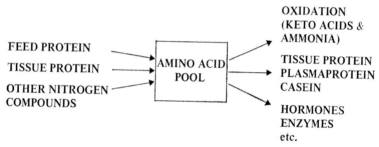

Fig.9.6. Amino acid metabolism.

The first step in the breakdown of amino acids involves transfer or removal of amino groups. Transamination reactions are conversions of one amino acid to the corresponding keto acid with simultaneous conversion of another keto acid to an amino acid. Oxidative deamination is a process by which an amino acid is converted to an imino acid, and this compound is hydrolyzed to the corresponding keto acid, with the liberation of ammonia. Amino acids can also take up ammonia, forming the corresponding amine. The nitrogen free residues of the deaminated amino acids are oxidized to carbon dioxide and water. Part of the energy released is stored in high energy bonds.

Most of the ammonia formed by deamination of amino acids is converted to urea which is excreted in the urine. The basic compounds required for urea synthesis are 2 moles of ammonia and 1 mole of carbon dioxide. The synthesis via the urea cycle involves conversion of the amino acid ornithine to citrulline and then to arginine, following which urea is split off and ornithine is regenerated.

Metabolism of lipids

The biologically important lipids are the triglycerides, the phospholipids, and the sterols. The lipids in the animal body are in a dynamic state of constant catabolism and anabolism. The lipids in cells are of two main types: structural lipids, mainly found in the cell membranes, and neutral fat, stored as energy reserves in the adipose cells of the fat depots.

Blood plasma contains about 300 mg lipids per 100 ml. About 50 per cent of this is phospholipids, about 30 per cent triglycerides, and 20 per cent cholesterol. Besides these major fractions the plasma contains small amounts of non-esterified fatty acids (NEFA). The NEFA have a very rapid turnover rate, and represent the main form in which fatty acids are transferred from fat depots to the site of oxidation. The oxidation of fatty acids takes place in the mitochondria by a process known as beta-oxidation. By this process the fatty acids are broken down to acetyl-Co-enzyme A, which enters the citric acid cycle and is oxidized to carbon dioxide and water. The energy released by this oxidation is stored as high energy bonds of ATP.

Many tissues can synthesize fatty acids from acetyl-CoA. Only small amounts of 12- and 14-carbon acids are formed, and none are synthesized with more than 16-carbon atoms. The pathway for fatty acid synthesis is not simply a reverse of the pathway for fat oxidation. The process involves the formation of malonyl-CoA by carboxylation of acetyl-CoA, and the combination of malonyl-CoA and acetyl-CoA.

Metabolism of carbohydrates

Part of the absorbed glucose is stored as glycogen in the liver. Liver glycogen represents an energy reserve that can be readily mobilized when required. The concentration of glucose in the mammalian blood plasma varies between 100 and 120 mg per 100 ml in simple stomached animals and between 40 and 60 mg per 100 ml in ruminants. The utilization of glucose requires its transport into the intracellular space where it is phosphorylated to form glucose-6-phosphate. This compound undergoes a series of chemical reactions to form pyruvic acid (Fig.9.7).

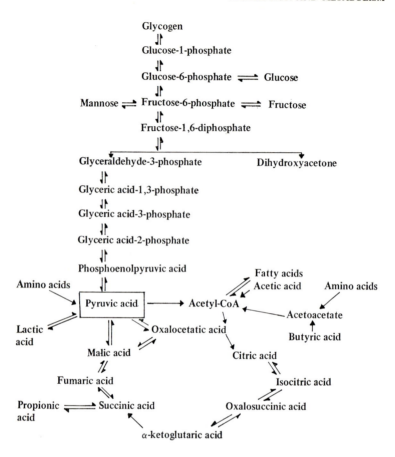

Fig.9.7. The biochemical pathways of carbohydrate metabolism and their combinations with protein and lipid metabolism.

In the presence of oxygen all cells except erythrocytes will oxidize pyruvic acid to carbon dioxide and water. This oxidation takes place through a chain of reactions known as the citric acid cycle. The first step involves the oxidative decarboxylation of pyruvic acid to acetyl-CoA, followed by the condensation of one mole of acetyl-CoA and one mole of oxalocetate to form one mole of citric acid. Through a number of oxidations and decarboxylations, the citric acid is broken down to oxalocetate.

The citric acid cycle is of equal importance in the metabolism of carbohydrate, lipid, and the nitrogen-free component of amino acids. It is the common reaction pathway for the metabolism of the nitrogen free energy releasing nutrients.

In ruminants the carbohydrates are fermented to acetic, propionic, and butyric acids in the rumen. These acids are absorbed from the rumen and serve in the energy metabolism. No glucose is absorbed in the ruminants. As seen in Fig. 9.7, acetic acid enters the metabolic pathways as acetyl-CoA, and may therefore be utilized in the synthesis of fat (high fat percentage in the milk). Butyric acid enters as acetoacetate and may also be utilized in fat synthesis. These two acids are ketogenic. Propionic acid enters the citric acid cycle as succinic acid, and may therefore be utilized in the synthesis of glucose and glycogen via the reaction malic acid $\rightleftharpoons$ pyruvic acid. Propionic acid is said to be glucogenic.

During both anaerobic and aerobic carbohydrate metabolism the released energy is taken up into the energy rich phosphate bonds in ATP. It can be calculated that 38 phosphate bonds are produced during the entire breakdown of one mole of glucose. The overall reaction will then be:

$$C_6H_{12}O_6 + 6O_2 + 38H_3PO_4 \rightarrow 6H_2O + 6CO_2 + 38ATP$$

The hydrolysis of one phosphate bond in ATP yields 10–12 kcal which means that for each mole of glucose metabolized about 420 kcal are produced. The energy of glucose is about 680 kcal per mole, so the degree of utilization is:

$$\frac{420}{680} \times 100 = 62 \text{ per cent}$$

The remaining 38 per cent disappears as heat.

10

Blood

Like other tissues, blood consists of cells and inter-cellular material. Unlike most tissues, however, the intercellular material is a fluid called plasma, and the cells are separate and free to move about within the vascular system. Some blood cells, the leukocytes, may even migrate through vessel walls to combat infections. The normal total circulating blood volume is about 8 per cent of the body weight.

The major functions of blood are: (1) transport of nutrients from the digestive tract to the body tissues; (2) transport of oxygen and carbon dioxide between lungs and body tissues; (3) transport of metabolic waste products from the body tissues to the kidneys; (4) transport of hormones from glands to other organs of the body; (5) regulation of acid-base and electrolyte balance of the body; (6) regulation of the body temperature; (7) defence against disease.

The specific gravity of blood is 1·040 to 1·050. It contains approximately 80 per cent water, 20 per cent organic matter, and less than 1 per cent inorganic matter. The colour varies according to the oxygen content. Oxygen-rich arterial blood has a pure red colour, whereas oxygen-poor venous blood has a dark red to brownish colour.

The hydrogen ion concentration of blood is very stable. In mammals the pH varies between 7·3 and 7·5. In birds the pH is about 7·6. The osmotic pressure is about 7 atmospheres due to salts. The osmotic pressure arising from proteins, known as the colloid oxmotic pressure, is only 20–25 mmHg, but of great importance for the exchange of fluid across the capillary wall (see Chapter 1). A 0·9 per cent sodium chloride solution has about the same osmotic pressure as blood and is said to be isotonic to blood.

CELLULAR COMPONENTS

The cellular components of the blood include red blood cells, white

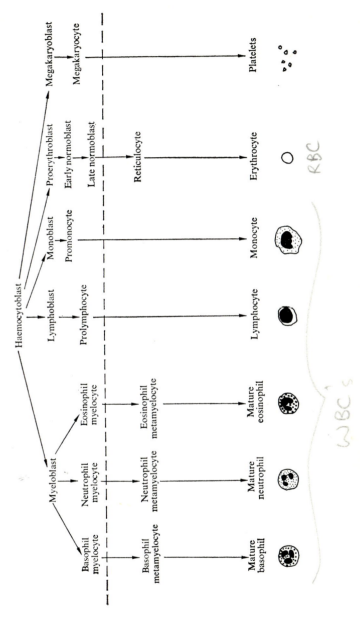

Fig.10.1. The synthesis of the blood cells. All those below the dotted line are normally found in peripheral blood while those above the line are normally found in the bone marrow (from Horrobin, *Medical Physiology and Biochemistry*, by kind permission of the author and Edward Arnold, 1968).

blood cells, and blood platelets. Because the red cells and the platelets both lack nuclei, they are not typical cells but might more appropriately be considered as portions of cells.

The red blood cells, or erythrocytes, carry haemoglobin in the circulation, and are therefore specialized for transport of oxygen. The erythrocytes are biconcave discs having a thick circular margin and a thin centre. They lose their nuclei before entering the circulation, and remain there for about 120 days.

The formation of red blood cells, erythropoiesis, takes place in the red bone marrow. In the foetus the cells are also formed in the liver. The formation is a continuous process that equals the rate of destruction. The rate of formation is regulated by a feed-back control which is inhibited by a rise in the circulating red cell level and stimulated by anaemia and lack of oxygen (hypoxia). Erythropoeisis is controlled by a hormone called erythropoietin, which is secreted by the kidneys.

Destruction of the red cells occurs after three to four months in circulation. The cells disintegrate and are removed from circulation by the reticuloendothelial system, which consists of special cells in the liver, spleen, bone marrow, and lymph nodes. Some of the products formed by red cell destruction include the bile pigments bilirubin and biliverdin, which are secreted by the liver into the bile. The released iron is used for resynthesis of haemoglobin.

The red oxygen carrying pigment in the red blood cells is haemoglobin, a protein with a molecular weight of about 68 000. The molecule is made up of four sub-units, each of which contains a haem moiety conjugated to a polypeptide. The presence of haemoglobin within the erythrocyte is responsible for its ability to carry oxygen and for the red colour of the cell. The haemoglobin absorbs oxygen from the air of the lungs to form oxyhaemoglobin, a loose combination which in turn readily gives up its oxygen to the tissue cells within the body.

$$Hb_4 + 4O_2 \rightleftharpoons Hb_4O^8$$

Because of the presence of haemoglobin, blood can carry about 60 times as much oxygen as a similar quantity of water under the same conditions. The process requires the presence of the Fe^{++} ion in the haemoglobin molecule. The combined oxygen is proportional to the amount of Fe^{++} present, with two atoms of oxygen united with each atom of iron. Each gram of haemoglobin will absorb 1·36 cm³ of oxygen. When the blood reaches tissues deficient in oxygen, the loosely held oxygen of the oxyhaemoglobin is given up readily, again forming reduced haemoglobin.

Methaemoglobin is a true oxidation product of haemoglobin which is unable to transport oxygen because the iron is in the ferric (Fe^{+++}) rather than the ferrous (Fe^{++}) state. Formation of methaemoglobin in cattle may be a result of nitrate poisoning in animals grazing newly fertilized fields.

Carboxyhaemoglobin is a stable compound formed when carbon monoxide (exhaust fumes) unites with haemoglobin. Since the affinity of CO is about 250 times that of O_2, a CO concentration of 0·1 per cent in the air represents a great danger to the organism.

The concentration of haemoglobin in the blood is between 10 and 15 g per 100 ml. When the concentration falls much below this value the animal is said to have developed anaemia. Anaemia may be due to deficient blood formation because of poor nutrition, including dietary deficiency of iron, copper, and vitamins. Anaemia may also be caused by loss of blood due to haemorrhage from wounds, or to parasites such as stomach worms or lice.

The white blood cells, or leukocytes, differ considerably from erythrocytes in that they are nucleated and possess independent movement. Leukocytes are classified as granulocytes and agranulocytes. The granulocytes are named according to the colour of the stained granules in the cells. Young granulocytes have horseshoe-shaped nuclei that become multilobular as the cells grow older.

Most of the granulocytes contain granules which can stain either blue or red with basic dyes and are known as neutrophils. They constitute the first line of defence against infection by migrating to any area invaded by bacteria, passing through vessel walls and engulfing the bacteria to destroy them. In the process many of the neutrophils also dissolve dead tissue in the area and the resulting semi-liquid material is known as pus.

A few leukocytes contain granules that stain with acid dyes. They are known as eosinophils. The number of these cells is quite small, but increases in case of infestation with parasites.

The basophil granulocytes contain blue staining granules. They are quite rare in normal blood.

The agranulocytes are lymphocytes and monocytes. The lymphocytes are important in forming barriers against local disease conditions and are involved in antibody formation in the development of immunity to disease.

The monocytes, like the neutrophils, are phagocytic. Their

number increases in case of chronic infections such as tuberculosis.

Thrombocytes or blood platelets are fragments of protoplasm about 2–4 μ in diameter. The thrombocytes contain considerable amounts of protein, lipids, enzymes, and minerals. Their life span is only 8–10 days, and they are formed in the bone marrow and in the spleen. The function of the platelets is chiefly to reduce loss of blood from injured vessels by acting in the coagulation of the blood.

Table 10.1 Approximate values for the blood content of leukocytes

Animal	Total no. ($10^3/mm^3$)	Distribution in %				
		Neutrophils	Eosinophils	Basophils	Lymphocytes	Monocytes
Horse	7–10	60	6	0·5	30	4
Cattle	5–12	35	8	0·1	53	4
Sheep	6–11	30	7	0·5	60	3
Goat	5–14	35	6	0·5	55	1
Pig	10–20	55	2	1·0	40	2

BLOOD PLASMA

The blood plasma makes up 60–65 per cent of the blood volume. It is a yellowish fluid. The specific gravity varies between 1·025 and 1·030 and is proportional to the plasma protein concentration. The organic contents are about 8–9 per cent and the inorganic about 1 per cent. The blood plasma contains 6–8 g per 100 ml protein of which 0·5 g per 100 ml is fibrinogen, 3·0–3·5 g per 100 ml is albumin, and 3·5–4·0 g per 100 ml is globulin. The globulin fraction may be divided into alpha-, beta-, and gamma-globulins. Blood plasma less fibrinogen is called blood serum.

The capillary walls are impermeable to the plasma proteins, and the proteins therefore exert an osmotic force of about 25 mmHg, known as the colloid osmotic pressure or the oncotic pressure. The force tends to pull water into the capillary (see Chapter 1). If the protein concentration falls below 3–4·6 per cent in the blood, the colloid osmotic pressure will be so low that water will not be pulled back into the venous end of the capillary, and oedema will result.

The plasma proteins are also responsible for part of the buffering capacity of the blood because of the weak ionization of the $-COOH$ and $-NH_2$ groups. At the normal plasma pH of 7·4, the proteins are in the anionic form and constitute a significant part of the anionic part of the plasma.

The plasma proteins are also of importance as carriers of anti-bodies (gamma-globulin), and as carriers of nutrients that are insoluble in water, such as fatty acids. Plasma proteins are mainly of the albumin fraction, also utilized in the synthesis of tissue proteins.

BLOOD CLOTTING

The initial reaction in blood clotting is the formation of a compound known as thromboplastin. This can be released either by damaged tissues or as the result of a complex series of reactions in the blood involving platelets (thrombocytes) and a whole series of clotting factors including anti-haemophilic factor. Calcium ions are required for the formation of thromboplastin from blood.

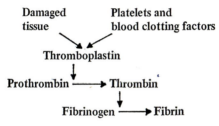

Fig.10.2. Outline of the process of blood clotting.

Thromboplastin is an enzyme which converts prothrombin which is present in the plasma to thrombin. Again calcium ions are required. Prothrombin and the clotting factors required for thromboplastin production are manufactured in the liver; vitamin K is essential for the process.

Thrombin then splits fibrinogen, another blood protein, to form the insoluble threads of fibrin. The fibrin threads, under the influence of substances released from platelets, contract together to form a firm clot (thrombus).

Because calcium ions are so important in blood clotting, the process can be prevented by removing the calcium ions from solution. This can be done by adding citrate, oxalate or EDTA to the blood. All three substances bind calcium ions.

Substances which block the action of vitamin K in the liver can also interfere with clotting. There are several substances, such as dicoumarol, which have this action. They occur naturally in some plants and were discovered when cattle in Canada developed a bleeding disease after feeding on a particular pasture.

LYMPH

Much of the fluid that passes through the capillary membrane into the tissue is reabsorbed. Excess tissue fluid is picked up by a system of blind capillaries called lymphatics. The fluid, known as lymph, is a clear, colourless liquid containing very little protein, but otherwise the same quantity of chemicals as the plasma.

Lymph which drains the intestine may contain large quantities of fat, and the lymph in the thoracic duct after a meal is milky because of its high fat content. The lymphocytes, produced in the lymph nodes, enter the circulation via the lymphatics. Eventually all lymph is returned to the venous blood via the thoracic and right lymphatic ducts.

BLOOD GROUPS IN MAN AND ANIMALS

Blood groups in man and animals are defined as the sum of all the serological antigens, blood group factors, attached to the membrane of the red blood cells. An antigen is a chemical compound, usually a protein, which when injected into an individual that lacks it, will cause the formation of a specific antigen neutralizing compound, the antibody. When the antigen is attached to the red blood cell, the antigen–antibody reaction may cause: (1) damage to the cell membrane and release of the haemoglobin, a process known as haemolysis, or (2) clumping of the cells known as agglutination, with subsequent haemolysis. In the blood plasma of some individuals antibodies against antigens from the red blood cells of other individuals are found, these are known as natural or preformed antibodies. If the blood from two such individuals is mixed the antigen–antibody reaction will occur. The blood groups can thus be determined by mixing red blood cells in an isotonic saline solution with serum from another individual whose antibody content is known. If haemolysis or agglutination occurs the particular blood group is present.

The blood group factors of different blood group systems are inherited independently of each other. Some systems have only one gene, or factor, whereas others have several. A single individual, however, can only possess two genes dealing with a particular group, one on each of the paired chromosomes contributed by its parents.

In humans the knowledge of blood groups allows the use of blood transfusions in medicine. Some diseases both in man and animals are caused by antigen–antibody reactions between the pregnant mother and the foetus. Because of the large number of blood groups, the number of combinations is very large. This allows the use of blood groups as means of identification. Finally because of the heredity of blood groups, these may be used to identify paternity. This is of medico-legal importance in humans, and of importance in animal breeding programmes.

Blood groups in man

About twenty different blood group systems are known in man. Of these the ABO and the rhesus systems are the most important.

Based upon antigen–antibody tests all humans can be divided into four groups according to the ABO blood group system: blood group A, blood group B, blood group AB, and blood group O (zero). In the plasma of an individual with blood group A the antibodies against group B are found, in an individual with group B anti-A is found, in an individual with group AB no antibodies are found against either A or B, and in individuals with group O both anti-A and anti-B are present.

Table 10.2 The ABO blood group system in man

Blood group (Phenotype)	Genotype	Antigen on red blood cell	Antibody in plasma
A	AA AO	A	anti-B
B	BB BO	B	anti-A
AB	AB	A + B	none
O	OO	none	anti-A anti-B

It appears from Table 10.2 that incompatibility may be due to: (1) the blood cells from the donor being agglutinated by the antibodies in the plasma of the recipient, or (2) the blood cells of the recipient being agglutinated by the plasma antibodies of the donor. The first is by far the most important, because the donor blood usually only amounts to a small part of the blood volume of the recipient. It thus appears that group O blood may be used for transfusion independently of the blood group of the recipient, and that a person with blood group AB may be an universal recipient. In practice, however, transfusions are always given with blood of the same blood group as that of the recipient.

Based on the rhesus system all humans can be divided into two groups, those that possess the rhesus antigen on their red blood cells, classified Rh+, and those who do not, classified Rh−.

If a blood transfusion from a Rh+ donor is given to a Rh− recipient the latter will produce antibodies against the rhesus factor, and subsequent transfusions may cause transfusion reactions.

In pregnant women the blood cells may cross the placenta. If the woman is Rh− and the fetus is Rh+, inherited from the father, the woman may produce antibodies against the rhesus factor of the foetus. At the end of the pregnancy these antibodies may pass from the mother to the foetus and cause haemolysis of the blood of the new born child which will suffer severe anaemia. This condition only occurs in a small number of pregnancies of Rh− women with Rh+ foetuses.

Blood groups in cattle

In cattle 10 different blood group systems are found, several of these with a large number of antigen factors. Some of these factors are specific to certain cattle races, for instance the Z′ factor of the A

Table 10.3 Blood groups in cattle (Moustgaard).

			Blood group system						
A	*B*	*C*	*FV*	*J*	*L*	*M*	*SU*	*Z*	*R′s′*
A	B	C_1, C_2	F	J	L	M_1, M_2	S,H′	Z	R′
D	G	E	V				U_1		S′
H	I	N_1					U		
Z′	K	R							
	O_1, O_2, O_3	W							
	P	X_1, X_2, X_3							
	Q	L							
	T_1, T_2								
	Y_1, Y_2								
	A_1, A_2								
	B′								
	D′								
	E'_1, E'_2, E'_3								
	I′								
	J′								
	K′								
	O′								
	Y′								

Blood group factors

system occurs in Zebu cattle and its descendants, such as Jersey cattle. The only known natural antibody is anti-J in the J system. Blood transfusions in cattle, therefore, seldom cause any reactions the first time. Later transfusions to the same animal, however, may cause antigen–antibody reactions because of antibodies formed after the first transfusion.

The practical application of blood groups in cattle is primarily for the determination of paternity. In breeding schemes it is often of importance to ensure that a certain calf has been sired by a certain bull, or rather if several possible fathers exist, to determine those that could not possibly be the father. To do so it is necessary to have blood samples from the calf, the mother cow, and all the possible fathers.

It appears from Table 10.4 that in the A system the calf has the factor A, and in the SU system the factor S. If the mother has none of these factors, then the calf must have them from the father. Bull 1 has none of these and may be excluded as the father of the calf, whereas bull 2 has both factors and cannot be excluded. It appears that the blood group analysis does not tell who the father is, but rather who may be excluded as the father.

The method can also be used to determine whether two calves are identical twins. Since such animals are identical genetically, they may be used for research and can replace the use of large groups.

Table 10.4 Paternity determination in cattle [see text] (from Moustgaard).

Animal					*Blood group system*					
	A	*B*	*C*	*FV*	*J*	*L*	*M*	*SU*	*Z*	*R′S′*
Bull 1	–/–	BGO/	C_1X_1	F/V	–/–	L/–	–/–	–/–	Z/–	R′/S′
Bull 2	A/–	B/	W/	F/V	–/–	–/–	–/–	S/U′	Z/–	R′/S′
Cow	–/–	BO_1/	W/	F/V	J/–	–/–	–/–	–/–	–/–	R′/S′
Calf	A/–	B/	W/	F/V	J/–	–/–	–/–	S/–	Z/–	R′/S′

Blood group in pigs

Ten blood group systems are known in pigs. The number of factors is less than in cattle. As in cattle, blood group analysis in pigs is used to determine paternity.

In piglets a disease is known where the animals develop haemolytic anaemia when they start suckling the sow. This is due to antibodies in the milk reacting to antigens in the piglets blood. These antibodies are formed in the sow because antigens pass from the foetus to the sow during pregnancy. The antigens do not occur in the sow, but the foetuses have inherited them from the boar. A similar disease is found in foals.

11

Cardiovascular system

The cardiovascular system consists of a four-chambered pump, the heart, and a system of vessels in which the blood circulates. Vessels which carry blood away from the heart are arteries, those which carry blood towards the heart are veins. In addition, there is a system of vessels carrying tissue fluid or lymph to the large veins. These vessels known as lymph vessels, or lymphatics.

The heart allows the blood to flow only in one direction, entering the atria, passing to the ventricles, and leaving via the aorta or the pulmonary artery. The blood passes from the atria to the ventricles because the atria beat first followed by the ventricles. If an artery is cut the blood will spurt away from the heart, whereas the blood from a cut vein will dribble out towards the heart. This demonstrates that the blood flows from the arteries via the veins to the heart. The veins have valves which permit flow only towards the heart. Between the arteries and the veins are found the capillaries in which the exchange between blood and tissues takes place.

THE HEART

The heart consists of four chambers. The blood from the peripheral areas of the body, apart from the lungs, returns to the thin-walled right atrium. From here it passes to the right ventricle, which ejects it into the pulmonary circulation. The pulmonary veins return the blood to the left atrium from where it passes to the powerful left ventricle which finally ejects it into the aorta.

Heart muscle is striated, but exhibits several features which differentiate it from skeletal muscle. It is composed of branching fibres which appear at first to be linked in the form of a huge syncytium. However, at regular intervals, barriers known as inter-

5

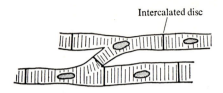

Intercalated disc

Fig.11.1. Cardiac muscle fibres (from Horrobin, *Medical Physiology and Biochemistry*, by kind permission of the author and Edward Arnold, 1968).

calated discs cross the fibres. They represent cell boundaries. Though not an anatomical syncytium, the heart behaves as a unit.

The heart is innervated from the sympathetic and the parasympathetic nervous system. The parasympathetic nerves go to the ganglia cells near the sino-atrial and atrio-ventricular nodes. From the ganglia, fibres go to the nodes and to the heart muscle. The sympathetic nerves follow the arteries in the heart to reach all muscle cells.

The neuromuscular system in the heart is composed of special muscle fibres, completely isolated from the rest of the heart muscle by connective tissue. The sino-atrial node is found in the wall of the right atrium near the ostium of the vena cava cranialis. The atrio-

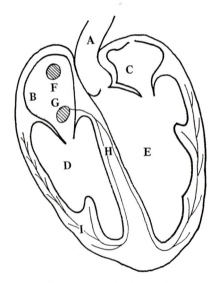

Fig.11.2. The neuromuscular system of the heart. (A) Aorta. (B) Right atrium. (C) Left atrium. (D) Right ventricle. (E) Left ventricle. (F) Sino-atrial node. (G) Atrio-ventricular node. (H) His bundle. (I) Purkinje fibres.

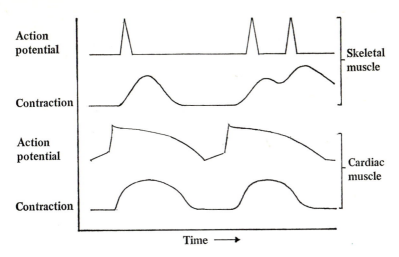

Fig.11.3. Comparison of the properties of cardiac and skeletal muscle (see text).

ventricular node is located in the septum between the two atria. There is no specialized conducting tissue between the two nodes, but the atrio-ventricular node continues in the bundle of His and the Purkinje fibres which reach the muscle cells of both ventricles (see Fig.11.2.).

The resting membrane potential of the cardiac muscle cells is about −80 mV with the interior negative to the exterior. Stimulation produces a propagated action potential which is responsible for initiating contraction. The regulation of the heart beat by the sino-atrial node, the atrio-ventricular node, the His bundle, and the Purkinje fibres is adequate to keep the heart beating regularly without outside nervous control. However, the rate of heartbeat and strength of contraction are regulated by impulses from the autonomic nervous system. Stimulation of the vagal nerve tends to inhibit the action of the heart by slowing the rate of beating of the sino-atrial node and the rate of conduction of impulses within the heart. Sympathetic stimulation increases activity of the heart by increasing the force of contraction, the rate of contraction, the rate of impulse conduction, and coronary blood flow.

The very long action potential and refractory period in cardiac muscle are of great importance. They ensure that, in contrast to the situation in skeletal muscle, two successive contractions cannot add together without a period of relaxation between them. The period of

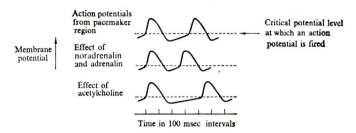

Fig.11.4. Action potential from the region of the sino-atrial node showing the instability of the drifting membrane potential and the action of acetylcholine and adrenalin (from Horrobin, *Medical Physiology and Biochemistry*, by kind permission of the author and Edward Arnold, 1968).

relaxation is essential to allow the heart to fill with blood. Without the long refractory period the heart could not function as a pump.

Recordings of the action potential and contraction in skeletal and heart muscle show the following differences (Fig.11.3): (1) in skeletal muscle the action potential is brief, lasting only about 1 msec. The action potential is initiated by a nervous impulse and afterwards the membrane potential returns to its original level and stays there until another nervous impulse appears. The contraction lasts very much longer than the action potential and the fibre is usually excitable again long before the contraction has even reached its peak (2). In cardiac muscle, no nervous impulse is required for the initiation of an action potential (3). Like the skeletal muscle action potential, that of the heart rises rapidly. However, the cardiac fibre remains depolarized and unexcitable for 150–500 msec. During this time the contraction rises to a peak and fades away. Only after the completion of the contraction does the membrane become repolarized. (4) After an action potential the cardiac membrane potential returns to about − 80 mV, but it does not stay there. It is unstable and drifts towards zero. When a critical level of depolarization is reached, another action potential is initiated. (5) The rate of drift is fastest in the region of the sino-atrial node and slowest in the ventricles. Thus the heart follows the rhythm of the sino-atrial node. (6) Acetylcholine reduces the rate of drift and thus slows down the rate of beating, whereas adrenalin increases the rate of drift and speeds up the heart (Fig.11.4).

The electrocardiogram (ECG) is a recording of the action potentials of the heart. Since the action potentials of the heart muscle do not occur synchronously over the whole heart, currents flow from one part to another in the extracellular fluid. These currents are conducted throughout the body and can be detected on the body surface by sensitive electrodes. The shape of the electrocardiogram can give information on certain diseases in the heart of man, and to some extent in animals.

The cardiac cycle

It is important to note that there are no valves guarding the entries to the atria. They are therefore ineffective pumps. The operation of the heart valves depends entirely on the pressure differences across them.

The period during which the heart contracts once is called the systolic period. It can be divided into two periods, pre-systole and systole. Pre-systole is the time from the beginning of the atrial contraction to the beginning of the ventricular contraction. Systole is the period from the beginning of the ventricular contraction to the end of the ventricular contraction. The systolic period is followed by a period where both atria and ventricles are relaxed. This period is known as diastole.

The pressure changes in the heart can be measured by means of catheters introduced into the heart through veins or arteries. The following description is of the left side of the heart. The right side does not differ in any important respect.

As the ventricle relaxes after its last beat, the pressure within it falls to below the pressure of the atrium. The atrio-ventricular valve opens and blood rushes into the ventricle. As the ventricle becomes full, the rapid filling is followed by a contraction of the atrium forcing a little extra blood into the ventricle. Because of the delay at the atrio-ventricular node, the ventricle contracts well after the atrium. As soon as the ventricular contraction begins, pressure rises in the ventricle, the atrio-ventricular valve closes and the filling phase ends. The contraction raises the pressure inside the ventricle, but cannot expel any blood until the aortic valve opens. This happens when the ventricular pressure rises above that of the aorta. Blood then rushes into the aorta faster than it can run out via the peripheral circulation. The pressure in the aorta thus rises, the ventricle relaxes, and the flow rate falls. Since the aortic pressure falls more rapidly than the ventricular, the valve remains open and ejection continues, but at a slower rate. Finally, however, the ventricular pressure drops below that in the aorta and the valve closes. The contraction is followed by relaxation of the whole heart and opening of the atrio-ventricular valve (Fig.11.5).

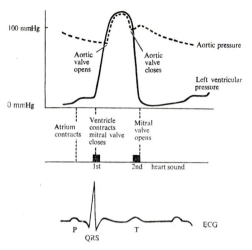

Fig.11.5. The main events of the cardiac cycle for the left side of the heart where the atrio-ventricular valve is known as the mitral valve. Events on the right side are essentially similar although the pressures involved are much lower (Horrobin).

Nourishment of the heart

The heart muscle receives blood through the two coronary arteries, extending from the aorta immediately after the semilunar valves. The veins of the coronary system open into the right atrium. The amount of blood that enters the coronary system depends on the aortic pressure. In the resting animal 3–5 per cent of the blood ejected from the heart enters the coronary circulation. Physical exercise increases this amount considerably.

Regulation of heart function

The volume of blood pumped out by one ventricle in one minute is defined as the cardiac output. It is equal to the product of the stroke volume and the heart rate. The output from the two ventricles must be equal, otherwise blood would pile up either in the lungs or in the body.

The heart function is regulated by the autonomic nervous system. Impulses in the vagal cardiac nerve fibres decrease heart rate. There is little tonic discharge in the cardiac sympathetic nerves, whereas there is a considerable tonic vagal discharge. If the vagal fibres to the heart are cut, the inhibitory impulses are removed and the heart rate increases.

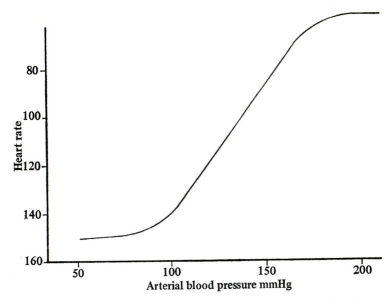

Fig.11.6. The relationship between blood pressure and frequency of heart beat.

In the walls of the aorta and the carotic artery the baroreceptors are found. These receptors are stimulated by distension of the arterial wall, and so they discharge at an increased rate when the blood pressure increases. The afferent nerves from the baroreceptors pass to the cardioinhibitory centre. Impulses generated in the baroreceptors thus excite the cardioinhibitory centre producing a decreased heart rate and a fall in blood pressure. An increase in the arterial blood pressure will in this way reflexly decrease the frequency of the heart rate, whereas a fall in arterial blood pressure causes an increase in heart rate (Fig.11.6).

PERIPHERAL CIRCULATION

The blood vessels are a closed system of tubes which carry blood from the heart to the tissues and back to the heart. The vessels consist of arteries, arterioles, capillaries, venules, veins, and in some regions arteriovenous anastomoses. All these vessels, with the possible exception of capillaries, are under nervous or hormonal control.

The large arteries have mainly elastic walls, whereas in the arterioles the smooth muscle layer is more pronounced. The muscle cells disappear gradually in the capillaries, which appear as thin endothelial tubes. The Rouget cells, found on the outside of the endothelial cells are believed to have a function similar to that of muscle cells.

The smooth muscles in the large arteries play no role in normal physiology, but are very important following damage to the artery. Provided that the damage is not too great, spasm of the smooth muscles may succeed in closing it and stop the bleeding.

The arterioles are all supplied with sympathetic nerve fibres, whereas there is no evidence of a parasympathetic nerve supply to the arterioles. The sympathetic fibres are tonically active, releasing a steady stream of noradrenalin causing the arterioles to remain partially constricted. A reduction in the sympathetic discharge will lead to dilatation, and an increase to further constriction.

Observations of the capillaries reveal that for a short period all the capillaries of a certain area are full of blood. Then, for no apparent reason, they empty and a moment later they fill again. It has not been proved whether these variations in capillary filling are due to active capillary constrictions or are merely a consequence of change in the arterioles.

Relatively little is known about the control of the veins and venules. Their smooth muscle is well supplied with sympathetic vasoconstrictor nerves and they may also contract in response to circulating adrenalin.

Principles of circulation

If the pressure under which the blood passes to the different parts of the circulatory system is measured, the following values are found: aorta 180–100 mmHg, arterioles 80–40 mmHg, capillaries 30–10 mmHg, veins 10–1 mmHg, and in the central veins a slightly negative pressure owing to the influence of the negative pressure in the thoracic cavity.

The relationship between flow, pressure, and resistance in the blood vessels can be expressed in the following way:

$$\text{Flow} = \frac{\text{Pressure}}{\text{Resistance}}$$

Blood always flows from areas of high pressure to areas of low pressure (Fig.11.7), and the flow in any part of the vascular system is equal to the effective perfusion pressure in that part divided by the

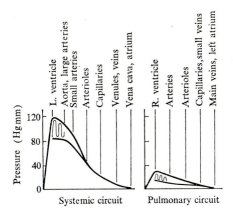

Fig.11.7. Approximate values for pressures in various parts of the circulatory system (from Horrobin, *Medical Physiology and Biochemistry*, by kind permission of the author and Edward Arnold, 1968).

resistance. The effective perfusion pressure is the mean intraluminal pressure at the arterial end minus the mean pressure at the venous end.

When the left ventricle pumps a surge of blood out into the aorta during systole, the blood cannot leave the aorta and main arteries as quickly as it is pumped in. Because the aorta and arteries have elastic walls, they therefore become stretched and expand. During diastole, when the heart is not pumping blood, the elastic recoil of the aorta and arteries causes them to contract and thus to maintain the flow of blood and the blood pressure.

The highest pressure in the arteries occurs during systole, the systolic blood pressure, and the lowest pressure occurs during diastole, the diastolic blood pressure. Increased blood pressure may be caused by decreased elasticity of the arteries or by increased sympathetic discharge causing constriction of the arterioles and thereby increased resistance. Increased blood pressure will cause enlargement of the heart.

Each systolic contraction of the left ventricle forces more blood into the arterial bed, which is already filled with blood under considerable pressure. This additional blood both dilates and lengthens the elastic arteries and forces more blood into the capillaries. The wave of increased systolic pressure which starts in the heart and spreads throughout the arteries to the capillaries is called the pulse wave.

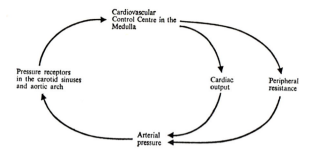

Fig.11.8. The control of arterial pressure (Horrobin).

Only a small part of the arterial blood pressure carries through the capillary bed to assist the return of the blood to the heart. None of this pressure affects the return of lymph to the venous circulation. Of major importance for venous return are the valves found in both the veins and lymph vessels. These valves permit movement of fluid in only one direction. Therefore, anything that applies pressure to a segment of a vein or lymph vessel acts as a pump and moves the fluid towards the heart. Muscular movements thus force the fluid out of a segment of the vein in the direction of the heart.

Contraction of the diaphragm during respiration also aids the movement of blood and lymph. When the diaphragm contracts the negative pressure in the thoracic cavity is increased and the blood is sucked from the abdominal veins into the thoracic veins.

REGULATION OF BLOOD CIRCULATION

In mammals several regulatory mechanisms for the cardiovascular system have evolved. These mechanisms increase the blood supply to active tissues and increase or decrease the heat loss from the body by redistributing the blood. The circulatory adjustments are effected by neural and chemical mechanisms that change the calibre of the arterioles, increase or decrease blood storage in venous reservoirs, and vary the rate and stroke output of the heart.

Chemical changes in active tissues dilate the arterioles by direct action on their smooth muscle. Decreased oxygen tension and pH cause vasodilatation, as does a rise in carbon dioxide tension. A rise in temperature due to the heat of metabolism exerts a direct vasodilatory effect. Another substance which accumulates locally and may have a vasodilatory effect is lactic acid.

Local vasoconstriction is seen in injured vessels. The constriction appears to be due to the local liberation of substances from the platelets which stick to the vessel wall in the injured area.

Noradrenalin and adrenalin are vasomotor agents frequently found in the circulating blood. Noradrenalin has a generalized vaso-constrictor action, whereas adrenalin dilates the vessels in skeletal muscle.

Although the arterioles are most densely innervated, all blood vessels except capillaries contain smooth muscle and receive motor nerve fibres from the sympathetic nervous system. The fibres to the arterioles regulate tissue blood flow and arterial pressure by altering the resistance in the arterioles. The fibres to the venous vessels vary the volume of blood stored in the veins. The constriction of the veins is produced by stimuli which strongly activate the vasoconstrictor nerves to the arterioles. The decrease in venous capacity increases the venous return to the heart, thus shifting the blood to the arterial side of the circulatory system.

The receptor mechanisms for detecting the arterial blood pressure are found in the walls of the carotid sinuses and the aortic arch. These receptors, known as baroreceptors, are stimulated by dis-tension. This stimulation causes discharge at an increased rate which, via the central nervous system, stimulates various effector mech-anisms. The impulses from the baroreceptors inhibit the tonic dis-charge of the vasoconstrictor nerves, producing dilatation of the arterioles, and excite the cardioinhibitory centre, causing a fall in the heart rate. The overall result of the baroreceptor stimulation is a fall in the blood pressure to a normal level.

When the blood pressure falls below a certain level the discharge from the baroreceptors falls. This stimulates the vasoconstrictor nerves, causing a rise in arterial blood pressure and an increased venous return. Furthermore, the cardiac centre becomes less in-hibited and the heart rate rises owing to a fall in vagal activity and a rise in sympathetic activity (Fig.11.8).

12

Respiratory system

MECHANISM OF BREATHING

The major function of the respiratory system is the movement of oxygen from the outside air to the lungs and the movement
of carbon dioxide in the reverse direction. Respiration furthermore
involves the transfer of these gases from the lungs to the blood and
vice versa. These processes involve a combination of lung function
and pulmonary blood circulation.

After passing through the nasal passages and the pharynx, where
it is warmed and takes up water vapour, the inspired air passes down
the trachea and through the bronchioles, respiratory bronchioles, and
alveolar ducts to the alveoli. The alveoli are surrounded by pulmonary capillaries, and the structures between the air and the
capillary blood are normally very thin. The total area of the alveolar
walls in contact with capillaries is very large, in humans about
70–90 m².

The lungs lie within the chest and are very elastic structures. When
taken out of the chest they collapse and occupy a very small volume.
In life, of course, they are expanded but, contrary to what one
might expect, they are not attached to the chest wall by any actual
tissue connections.

The lungs are covered by a very smooth, moist membrane known
as the visceral pleura. The chest wall is lined by a similar smooth
moist membrane known as the parietal pleura. In normal individuals
these two layers are closely applied to one another. Although there
are no actual bridges of tissue between them, the two layers never
normally come apart. When the chest wall expands, the visceral
pleura is pulled outwards in company with the parietal pleura and
the visceral pleura in turn pulls out the underlying lungs. The
pleural cavity is the space between the two pleural layers. Normally

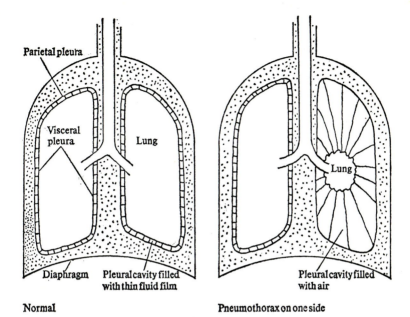

Parietal pleura

Visceral pleura

Lung

Diaphragm

Pleural cavity filled with thin fluid film

Normal

Lung

Pleural cavity filled with air

Pneumothorax on one side

Fig.12.1. The lungs and pleural membranes showing how a pneumothorax can occur (Horrobin).

it contains nothing but a very thin layer of liquid and is thus more of a potential space than a real one.

The only link between the two moist pleural surfaces is a thin film of water. Because of the force of surface tension, the water molecules in the film strongly resist being pulled apart from one another. The same force can be easily demonstrated outside the body by using two microscope slides with a thin film of water between them. It is surprisingly difficult to pull the two slides apart because of surface tension. Sometimes, usually because of a chest injury, one or other of the pleural layers is torn and air gets into the cavity either from the lungs or from the outside. This breaks the link between the visceral and parietal pleura and the natural elasticity of the underlying lung causes it to collapse. This is known as a pneumothorax (Fig.12.1).

Inspiration is an active process brought about by contraction of the inspiratory muscles. The most important inspiratory muscle is the diaphragm, which is attached to the caudal margins of the thoracic cage. When relaxed, it is domed into the thorax. When the

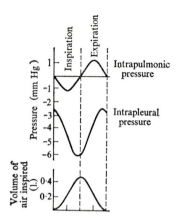

Fig.12.2. The changes in intrapleural and intrapulmonic (inside the lungs) pressure during inspiration and expiration (from Horrobin, *Medical Physiology and Biochemistry*, by kind permission of the author and Edward Arnold, 1968).

muscle fibres contract the diaphragm is pulled into a more straight position, thus increasing the volume of the thorax. The ribs are suspended from the vertebral column and attached either directly or indirectly to the sternum. If the ribs are raised, the diameter of the thorax will increase. This movement depends mainly on the internal and external intercostal muscles.

During quiet breathing the intrapleural pressure, which is about -2.5 mmHg (relative to atmosphere) at the start of inspiration, decreases to about -6 mmHg, and the lungs are pulled into a more expanded position. During expiration the intrapleural pressure returns to the original level. At the end of expiration, when no air movement occurs, the pressure in the bronchi is equal to atmospheric pressure. As the thorax expands, the lungs must expand also. Their volume increases, but initially the amount of air within them remains the same and so the pressure falls. This leads to a flow of air from the atmosphere into the lungs in order to equalize the pressures. When the flow into the lungs ceases at the end of inspiration, the intrapulmonic pressure is again equal to atmospheric pressure, while the intrapleural pressure is at its lowest. As the inspiratory muscles relax, the thoracic volume decreases, but the amount of air initially remains the same. The intrapulmonic pressure therefore rises above atmospheric pressure and so air flows from the lungs to the exterior until the pressures are equal again (Fig.12.2).

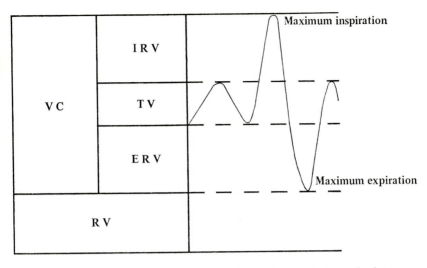

Fig.12.3. The relationship between the various volumes of air in the lungs. VC = vital capacity. IRV = inspiratory reserve volume. TV = tidal volume. ERV = expiratory reserve volume. RV = residual volume.

Respiration volume and frequency

Before reaching the alveoli, air must pass through the nose or mouth, pharynx, trachea, bronchi and bronchioles. The volume of gas in these tubes plays no part in gas exchange and so the volume of the airways is known as the anatomical dead space.

The volume of air which passes into or out of the nose and mouth during inspiration and expiration is known as the tidal volume. In horses it is about 5·6 1, in cattle 3·4 1, and in sheep and goats approximately 300 ml. The volume of the anatomical dead space is approximately a quarter to a third of the tidal volume. The volume of air which reaches the alveoli and which is available for exchange is equal to the tidal volume minus the anatomical dead space.

Various other air volumes are sometimes used in discussing respiration. Starting at the end of a quiet inspiration, the extra amount of air that can be inspired is the inspiratory reserve volume. Starting at the end of a quiet expiration, the extra amount that can be expired is the expiratory reserve volume. The vital capacity is the combined inspiratory reserve volume, the tidal volume, and the expiratory reserve volume. Even after a maximal expiration some air remains in the lungs, it is known as the residual volume (Fig. 12.3).

Table 12.1 The air volumes in the lungs of different animals [in litres]

Animal	Tidal volume	Inspiratory reserve volume	Expiratory reserve volume	Vital capacity	Residual volume
Horse	5–6	12	12	30	10–12
Cattle	3–4	6	6	16	5–6
Sheep	0·3	0·6	0·6	1·5	0·5
Man	0·5	1·5	1·5	4	1

Control of respiration

Spontaneous respiration is dependent upon the rhythmic discharge of the respiratory centre in the medulla oblongata. If the efferent nerves from the centre to the respiratory muscles are interrupted or the centre itself is destroyed, breathing stops. Changes in respiratory rates depend on changes in the rhythmic discharge.

The activity of the respiratory centre is regulated by changes in pCO_2, pO_2, and pH of the blood (p = partial pressure). Receptors capable of detecting these chemical changes in the blood are situated in the chemoreceptors, special cells found in the aortic arch and in the carotic sinuses. The chemoreceptors are stimulated by a rise in the pCO_2 or H^+ concentration of the arterial blood or by a decline in its pO_2.

In the resting animal the respiration rate is proportional to the pCO_2 of the blood in the range 35–60 mmHg. If the animal, for instance, has a venous pCO_2 of 45 mmHg and an arterial pCO_2 of 40 mmHg, the respiration remains constant. If the metabolism, and thereby the CO_2 production in the tissue is increased, the pCO_2 of the venous blood increases. This causes an increase in the pCO_2 of the air in the alveoles. The arterial blood therefore leaves the lungs with a higher pCO_2. This causes excitation of the respiratory centre and the respiration rate increases until normal arterial pCO_2 is restored. The opposite reaction occurs if the CO_2 production suddenly decreases.

A fall in the pH of the blood produces a pronounced respiratory stimulation. The hyperventilation decreases alveolar pCO_2 and thus produces a compensatory fall in blood H^+ concentration. Conversely, when blood pH rises, ventilation is depressed, and the arterial pCO_2 rises, raising the H^+ concentration to normal values

The relationship between pH and pCO_2 in blood is regulated by:

$$pH = pK + \log \frac{[HCO_3^-]}{pCO_2 \times 0.03} \quad \text{(See Chapter 1)}$$

When the O_2 content of the inspired air is decreased, there is an increase in respiration. The stimulation is marked when the pO_2 falls below 60 mmHg.

Exchange of oxygen and carbon dioxide between air and blood

The composition of atmospheric air is constant: 20·93 per cent by volume oxygen, 0·03 per cent carbon dioxide, and 79·04 per cent nitrogen. The inspiratory air has the same composition, whereas the expiratory air contains less oxygen and more carbon dioxide. The amount of nitrogen is unaltered.

Table 12.2 The oxygen, carbon dioxide, and nitrogen content of inspiratory, expiratory, and alveolar air

	Oxygen Vol.%	pO_2 (mmHg)	Carbon dioxide Vol.%	pCO_2 (mmHg)	Nitrogen Vol.%	PN_2 (mmHg)
Inspiratory air	20·9	159	0·03	0·23	79·0	600
Expiratory air	16·3	124	4·0	30	79·3	603
Alveolar air	14·0	106	5·3	40	74·5	567

The exchange of gases across the alveolar membrane is governed by two physical laws: (1) the amount of a gas bound physically in a liquid is proportional to the partial pressure of the gas (Henry's law); (2) individual gases are bound in the liquid independently of other gases (Dalton's law).

Table 12.3 The partial pressure of gases in blood and tissue of the resting animal

	pO_2	pCO_2	pN_2
Arterial blood	100	40	567
Venous blood	40–50	46	567
Tissue	20–40	50	567

By comparing tables 12.2 and 12.3 it is apparent that oxygen from the inspiratory air must pass to the venous blood in the lungs: pO_2 in the air is 159 and in the blood 50 mmHg. Since the pCO_2 of the venous blood is 46 and the pCO_2 of the inspired air is 0·23 mmHg, carbon dioxide will readily move from the blood to the air.

The gases are absorbed directly into the blood plasma, but only a small fraction of the gases is carried in physical solution in the fluid. Most of the oxygen is carried in combination with haemoglobin in the erythrocytes, and much of the carbon dioxide is carried in the bicarbonate form and as carbonic acid, and combined with haemoglobin as carbamino-haemoglobin.

Each gram of haemoglobin can combine with 1·36 ml oxygen. Since blood contains a little less than 15 grams of haemoglobin per 100 ml, 100 ml of fully oxygenated blood contains about 20 ml of oxygen. Blood leaving the lung capillaries is about 98 per cent saturated with oxygen.

The amount of oxygen that haemoglobin can carry is decreased by the presence of carbon dioxide, increased acidity, high temperature, and a low pO_2 in the surrounding medium.

The dissociation curve for oxygen from haemoglobin is hyperbolic in shape (Fig.12.4). The steep portion between pO_2 20–60 mmHg indicates that large amounts are given off to the tissues (see also table 12.3). The flat portion of the curve above pO_2 of 80 mmHg indicates that arterial blood has a nearly constant content of oxygen even though alveolar air may vary over a rather wide range of values. These characteristics encourage saturation of haemoglobin when blood is in contact with alveoli, yet they permit oxygen to be given off to tissues with a low pO_2.

Carbon dioxide produced by the tissues favours the release of oxygen from haemoglobin. The presence of carbon dioxide makes the blood more acid and the carbamino-haemoglobin which forms has less affinity for oxygen than normal haemoglobin. Therefore the blood will hold less oxygen, making more available for the tissues (Fig.12.4).

A higher temperature also favours the release of oxygen from haemoglobin. This is of importance because rapidly metabolizing cells have a high temperature and need more oxygen than inactive cells.

Carbon dioxide from the tissues enters the systemic capillaries because the pCO_2 of the tissue fluid is higher than the pCO_2 of the blood. At the same time oxygen diffuses across the capillary endo-

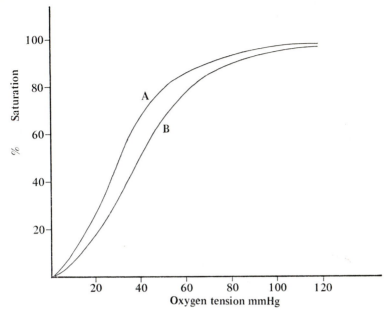

Fig.12.4. Oxygen dissociation curves under varying carbon dioxide tensions. (A) $pCO_2 = 40$ mmHg, (B) $pCO_2 = 80$ mmHg.

thelium in the opposite direction. About one fifth of the carbon dioxide appears to be combined with an amino group ($-NH_2$) in the form:

$$R-NH_2 + CO_2 \rightleftharpoons R-NH-COOH$$

Reduced haemoglobin is able to carry about three times as much carbamino bound carbon dioxide as oxygenated blood.

The remaining part of the carbon dioxide is carried by the blood as plasma bicarbonate. During increased pCO_2 carbon dioxide will diffuse into the red blood cells, where the following reaction is catalyzed by the enzyme carbonic anhydrase:

$$CO_2 + H_2O \rightleftharpoons H_2CO_3 \rightleftharpoons H^+ + HCO_3^-$$

The increase in intracellular bicarbonate concentration causes an exchange between bicarbonate and chloride from the plasma. The increased pCO_2 will thus cause an increase in plasma bicarbonate and a fall in plasma chloride (Fig.12.5).

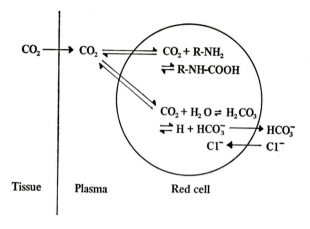

Fig.12.5. The principles of carbon dioxide transport between tissues and blood In the lungs reactions are reversed and carbon dioxide is excreted into the alveolar air and expired.

13

Urinary system

The urinary system is responsible for excretion of many waste products of the body. It is also an important factor in maintenance of homeostasis, the relative constant condition of the internal environment of the body. This includes regulation of water balance, acid-base balance, osmotic pressure, electrolyte levels, and levels of many other substances. This control is obtained by filtering a large quantity of water and other small molecules through the glomerulus. The appropriate amounts of each substance are then reabsorbed by the tubular cells, either passively by such forces as osmosis and diffusion, or actively.

ANATOMICAL STRUCTURE

The main gross anatomical features of the kidneys may be seen in a longitudinal section through the organ (Fig.13.1). The urine drains into the ureter from the large central cavity, the renal pelvis. The pelvis extends into the renal tissue by prolongations known as calyces. Cones of tissue, the renal papillae project, into the calyces. Opening on to the papillae are the tiny orifices of the ducts, formed by the fusion of several collecting ducts. The renal tissue is divided into an outer dark cortex, and an inner pale medulla.

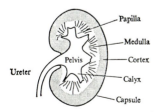

Fig.13.1. The main features of kidney structure seen in longitudinal section

The essential units of the kidneys are the blind ended tubes known as nephrons. The horse kidney contains about 2·5 million, the pig kidney about 1 million, and the sheep kidney about 0·5 million nephrons. The nephron consists of a single layer of epithelial cells surrounded by a basement membrane. At the blind ends, which lie in the cortex there is a cup, known as the Bowman's capsule. Immediately adjacent to the capsule is the convoluted part of the proximal tubule. This part continues in Henle's loop which dips down towards the medulla. This thin section of the nephron is U-shaped and continues back into the medulla, where the coils of the convoluted parts of the distal tubule are found in the region of the Bowman's capsule.

The Bowman's capsule contains the glomerulus, a complex network of capillaries. The glomerulus has arterioles at both ends. The afferent (incoming) arterioles are larger in diameter than the efferent (outgoing). (Fig.13.2).

The kidney has a rich sympathetic nerve supply. The nerves carry vasoconstrictor fibres to afferent and efferent arterioles.

FUNCTION

Filtration

The first step in urine formation takes place in the Bowman's capsule where fluid passes from the glomeruli into the capsule. The filtration depends on the hydrostatic pressure, the permeability of the membrane of the glomerulus, and the surface area of the glomerular

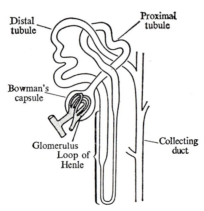

Fig.13.2. A nephron (from Horrobin, *Medical Physiology and Biochemistry*, by kind permission of the author and Edward Arnold, 1968).

capillaries. The hydrostatic pressure is determined by the degree of constriction of the afferent and efferent arterioles of the glomerulus. The membrane only allows molecules of a small size to pass. The capsule fluid therefore is protein-free, but otherwise contains the same ions and small molecules in the same concentration as that in which they are found in plasma within the limitations imposed by the Donnan equilibrium (see Chapter 1). The hydrostatic pressure in the glomerulus is approximately 70 mmHg. Acting against this, pressure is the hydrostatic pressure in the capsule, about 15 mmHg and the colloidal osmotic pressure of the blood, about 25 mmHg. The true filtration pressure is thus:

$$F = 70 - (15 + 25) = 30 \text{ mmHg}$$

As it is believed that all nephrons act simultaneously, it appears that variations in the glomerular filtration rate are mainly regulated by hydrostatic pressure in the glomerulus and only to a lesser degree by the filtration area.

Tubular function

Each day between 1000 and 2000 litres of fluid are delivered to the kidney tubules of the cow. This fluid contains large amounts of sodium, bicarbonate, glucose and other compounds. Since only between 10 and 20 litres of urine are excreted daily, the tubules must carry out the task of salvaging most of the material presented to them.

If a substance is moved from tubular fluid to blood, it is said to be reabsorbed. If it is moved from blood to tubular fluid, it is said to be secreted. Movements may be active as well as passive.

The amount of any substance that is filtered is the product of the rate of filtration in the glomerulus and the plasma concentration of the substance. The tubular cells may add more of the substance to the filtrate (tubular secretion), may remove some or all of the substance from the filtrate (tubular reabsorption), or may do both. The amount of the substance excreted is the concentration in the urine times urine volume. This amount equals the amount filtered plus the net amount transferred by the tubules (Fig.13.3).

Glomerular filtration rate

The glomerular filtration rate (GFR) can be determined by injecting into the blood stream a compound that is freely filtered at the

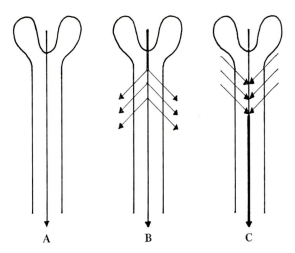

A.   Filtration, no
     reabsorption or secretion

B.   Filtration and
     reabsorption

C.   Filtration and
     secretion

Fig.13.3. Tubular function in the kidney (see text).

glomeruli but is neither reabsorbed nor secreted in the tubules. Since the concentration of such a substance will be the same in the plasma and in the glomerular filtrate, a blood sample can be used to determine its concentration in the glomerular filtrate.

This means that the total amount of substance X filtered per minute must equal the volume of the filtrate per minute (the GFR) multiplied by the concentration of X in the filtrate (or in the plasma).

Since X is neither reabsorbed nor secreted in the tubules, all that which is filtered will appear in the urine. Therefore the total amount filtered per minute will be equal to the volume of urine excreted per minute multiplied by the concentration of X in the urine.

Let P be the plasma concentration of X.
Let U be the urine concentration of X.
Let V be the urine volume per minute.
Let GFR be the volume of glomerular filtrate per minute.

Then total amount of X filtered $= \text{GFR} \times \text{P}$
$$\text{and also} = \text{U} \times \text{V}$$

$$\text{Therefore U} \times \text{V} = \text{GFR} \times \text{P}$$

$$\text{and GFR} = \frac{\text{U} \times \text{V}}{\text{P}}$$

The expression $\dfrac{\text{UV}}{\text{P}}$ is known as the clearance and is the volume of plasma which can be totally cleared of a substance per minute. With a substance like the polysaccharide inulin which is neither secreted nor reabsorbed, the clearance is equal to the GFR. If the clearance of a substance is found to be less than that of inulin, this indicates that it is reabsorbed in the tubules. If the clearance of a substance is more than that of inulin, the substance must be secreted into the tubules.

Mechanisms of tubular reabsorption and secretion

Water moves passively through the walls of the renal tubules down an osmotic gradient. Solute particles move passively into and out of the tubular fluid down chemical and electrical gradients, but many compounds are also actively transported against chemical and electrical gradients by energy requiring mechanisms. There is a maximal rate at which the renal active transport systems can transport a particular solute. The amount of a particular solute actively transported is thus proportionate to the amount present up to the maximum transport capacity. At higher concentrations the transport mechanism is saturated and there is no increment in the amount transported.

Glucose is typical of a substance removed from the urine by active transport. It is filtered at a rate of approximately 100 mg per min. The reabsorption occurs in the first part of the proximal tubule. Essentially all of the glucose is normally reabsorbed, and no more than a few mg appear in the urine per 24 hours. The amount reabsorbed is proportionate to the amount filtered and hence to the plasma glucose concentration up to the transport maximum, which is about 375 mg/min. The renal threshold for glucose is the plasma concentration at which the glucose first appears in the urine in more than the normal minute amounts (Figs.13.4 and 13.5).

The urine of mammals can be made hypertonic to blood. The majority of the fluid filtered from the glomerulus to the Bowman's

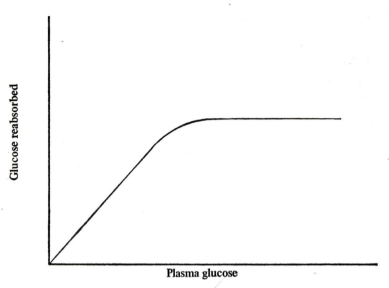

Fig.13.4. Relationship between plasma glucose level and amount of glucose reabsorbed.

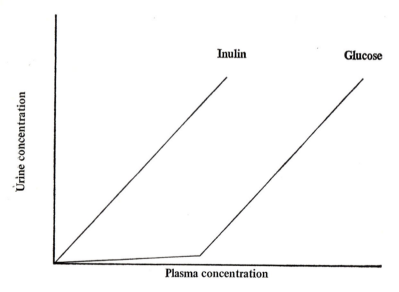

Fig.13.5. Relationship between plasma level and excretion of inulin and glucose in urine.

capsule is reabsorbed in the tubules, and the final urine volume amounts to 1–2 per cent of the filtrate.

It has been demonstrated that 80–90 per cent of the water in the filtrate is reabsorbed in the proximal tubule and in Henle's loop along an osmotic gradient. This is a result of the active movements of such compounds as sodium, potassium, glucose, chloride and bicarbonate. When the fluid leaves Henle's loop, it is still isotonic to blood, but the volume is reduced to about 10 per cent of the original filtrate. The remaining water absorption takes place in the distal tubules under influence of the antidiuretic hormone from the posterior lobe of the pituitary gland (see Chapter 5). In the presence of this hormone water is actively absorbed. If the hormone is absent, no water will be absorbed in the distal tubules and large volumes of urine are excreted. This condition is known as diabetes insipidus.

The clearance of urea is about 40 per cent of the inulin clearance. This means that 60 per cent of the urea filtered from the glomerulus has been reabsorbed in the tubules. If the animal is given less water, not only does the urine volume fall, but so also does urea clearance. This is of some importance in ruminants where the urea is recycled to the rumen via the saliva and utilized for the synthesis of microbial protein (see Chapter 8).

Hydrogen ions are secreted into both the proximal and distal tubules, mainly in exchange for the reabsorption of sodium ions. In the proximal tubule most of the hydrogen ions are buffered by combination with bicarbonate. When the bicarbonate has been used up as may often happen by the time the distal tubules are reached, the buffering is carried out by phosphate and by the secretion of ammonia (Fig. 13.6). The maximum acidity of the urine is about pH 4·5. At this point the hydrogen ion concentration in the urine is so high that no more hydrogen ions can be transported from the blood against the concentration gradient.

$$H^+ + HCO_3^- \rightleftharpoons H_2CO_3 \rightleftharpoons H_2O + CO_2$$

$$H^+ + HPO_4^= \rightleftharpoons H_2PO_4^-$$

$$H^+ + NH_3 \rightleftharpoons NH_4^+$$

Fig.13.6. The buffering of hydrogen ions in the urine.

When the plasma HCO_3^- concentration exceeds about 28 mEq/1, bicarbonate appears in the urine and urine becomes alkaline.

Sodium is filtered in large amounts, but is actively transported out of all portions of the tubules. Normally, therefore, 99 per cent of the filtered sodium is reabsorbed. Chloride reabsorption is increased when HCO_3^- reabsorption is decreased, and vice versa, so that the Cl^- concentration in the plasma varies inversely with the HCO_3^- concentration, keeping the total anion concentration constant. Much of the filtered potassium is removed from the tubular fluid by active reabsorption in the proximal tubules, and potassium is then secreted into the fluid by the distal tubular cells. In the absence of complicating factors, the amount secreted is approximately equal to the potassium intake and potassium balance is maintained.

MICTURITION

Micturition is the term for expulsion of urine from the bladder. It is a reflex activity stimulated by distension of the bladder from the constant inflow of urine by way of the ureters. The bladder adjusts to the gradual inflow of urine until the pressure becomes high enough to stimulate reflex centres in the spinal cord, which in turn causes contraction of the smooth muscle wall of the bladder by way of sacral parasympathetic nerves.

14

Reproduction

The primary reproductive organs in males are the testes. and in females they are the ovaries. The testes produce the male gametes or spermatozoa and the ovaries produce the female gametes or ova. In female mammals ovarian function is cyclic in nature and is associated with cyclic changes in behaviour and in other sex organs, notably the uterus. The uterine changes involve preparation for the reception of a fertilized ovum. If fertilization does not occur, the surface layers of the uterus atrophy in non-primates and are destroyed by bleeding (menstruation) in primates. In non-primates the female cycle is known as the oestrus cycle while in primates it is known as the menstrual cycle.

ROLE OF HORMONES IN THE REPRODUCTIVE PROCESS

After hypophysectomy (pituitary removal) in females, ovulation ceases, corpora lutea no longer form, follicles do not ripen and the ovary decreases in size. The interstitial cells undergo regressive changes: their nuclei become shrunken and the cytoplasm diminishes. The production of ovarian hormones, oestrogen and progesterone, is curtailed. Owing to lack of ovarian hormones, the dependent accessory organs (oviduct, uterus, vagina, and mammary glands) cease their rhythmical functional changes, decrease in size, and return to a structure closely resembling the infantile condition. If the female is immature at the time of the hypophysectomy the reproductive tract remains in the infantile condition.

In the male the same sequence of changes in the reproductive organs follows hypophysectomy. The testes rapidly atrophy and mature spermatozoa cease to be delivered to the epididymis. The interstitial cells between the tubules undergo regressive changes similar to those of the ovary. The accessory organs (prostate, seminal vesicles, and tubular pathways) deprived of the internal secretion from the interstitial cells, atrophy and in turn cease to secrete. If the operation is performed prior to maturity, testes and dependent reproductive organs fail to enlarge and differentiate, and never become functional.

Pituitary gonadotrophic complex

The gonadotrophically active substance in extracts from the anterior pituitary gland can be divided into two fractions. One fraction, when tested in immature female rats, causes growth of follicles. The follicles, however, do not progress to the formation of corpora lutea. The other fraction, although showing no gonadotrophic activity when given to normal immature rats, causes corpus luteum formation when combined with the first fraction. The active principle in the first fraction is called the follicle stimulating hormone (FSH), the second fraction the luteinizing hormone (LH). Given to the hypophysectomized male LH causes repair of the deficient interstitial cells of the testes. For this reason it has also been designated the interstitial cell stimulating hormone (ICSH).

Gonadal hormones

The gonads are the primary reproductive organs producing spermatozoa and ova. In addition to this the gonads are endocrine organs that produce and secrete steroids which regulate the reproductive functions. The hormones secreted by the gonads also regulate the development of the animal body and thus control the secondary sexual characteristics. In the young prepubertal animal the gonads secrete very small amounts of hormones. At puberty the gonads mature and start functioning. The age at which this occurs varies. In domestic animals the following ages in months can be given: horses 15–18, cattle 12–15, sheep and goats 8–12, and pigs 6–8.

The male sexual hormones are formed in the interstitial cells of the testes. Several steroids with androgen effect are produced, but the most important is testosterone. These hormones are responsible for the development of the sexual characteristics particular to the species. Prepubertal castration gives a clear negative picture of the action of the androgens. Penis, scrotum, and the secondary sexual organs fail to develop. The hormones also regulate the secretory activity of the prostate gland and the seminal vesicles. Removal of the pituitary gland causes atrophy of both the spermiogenetic tissue and the interstitial cells of the testes. The atrophy of the interstitial cells is caused by lack of ICSH, whereas the atrophy of the spermio-genetic tissue is caused by lack of androgens produced by the interstitial cells.

The androgens increase the rate of protein synthesis and retention of phosphate, potassium, sodium, and chloride.

The endocrine function of the testes is regulated by the interstitial stimulating hormone of the anterior lobe of the pituitary gland by means of a feed-back mechanism. Injection of androgens will inhibit the release of ICSH and cause atrophy of the testes, whereas a low androgen level in the blood stimulates the production of ICSH.

The female sexual hormones are produced in the ovary. Before the onset of puberty the production is low. When significant ovarian secretion commences it does so in a cyclic manner, continuing—apart from pregnancy or anoestrus—until the breeding age is past. There is a sudden increase in the size of the ovaries at puberty but the full development of the oestrus cycles is a gradual phenomenon preceded by incomplete cycles. This characterizes the period of adolescent sterility during which cyclic activity is accompanied by few fertile cycles. Thereafter full sexual maturity is gradually attained, although most animals are less than fully fertile at first. In pigs the first litter is generally smaller than subsequent ones and in sheep the proportion of singles at the first lambing is very high.

The oestrogens are produced in the cells lining the growing and mature follicles in the ovary. The effect of the oestrogens can be demonstrated by ovariectomy (surgical removal of the ovaries). The younger the age of ovariectomy, the more profound the results are likely to be. The operation results in failure of development of Fallopian tubes, uterus, vagina, and mammary glands. In the adult animal the oestrogens cause the epithelial cells in the vagina to proliferate and the cervix to open. The uterus varies according to the function of the ovary. In the juvenile animal the organ is small, the glands of the endometrium are not fully developed, and the myo-metrium is thin and shows no motility. Under influence of oestrogens the endometrial glands increase in size and the number of smooth muscle cells in the myometrium increases, and therefore also the motility.

Progesterone in the non-pregnant female is produced in the corpus luteum, which develops cyclically in the ovary. The hormone is normally released after a period of oestrogenic stimulation and many of its effects are not developed unless the animal has been primed with oestrogens in this manner. The most pronounced effects of progesterone are seen in the uterus. After a certain amount of response to oestrogen, when the endometrium undergoes proliferation, progesterone further enlarges the endometrial glands and causes them to secrete. Uterine motility is decreased, and the response of the uterus to oestrogen and to oxytocin is abolished.

During pregnancy there is a continuation of the progesterone phase of the oestrus cycle. Progesterone is essential for the maintenance of pregnancy in all its stages, and its withdrawal is followed by abortion or premature birth. The source of progesterone during pregnancy varies in different species, being mainly ovarian in the early stage and mainly placental in the later stage of pregnancy in most domestic animals.

Regulation of ovarian function

The hormonal secretion of the ovary is regulated by follicle stimulating hormone and luteinizing hormone, both released from the anterior lobe of the pituitary gland.

If FSH is injected into an infantile female the ovary will enlarge and small follicles will develop. The follicles, however, will not produce oestrogens unless LH is also present. LH furthermore regulates the development of the corpus luteum and the production of progesterone. As the follicle releases increasing amounts of oestrogen, FSH production is inhibited by this oestrogen, which simultaneously in some manner enhances LH production. When the correct ratio of FSH and LH is reached ovulation occurs and the corpus luteum is formed. The increase of progesterone in the blood inhibits the production of LH and thus increases the output of FSH.

In some animals ovulation will only occur following copulation. In rabbits ovulation occurs about 10 hours after copulation, which indicates a nervous link. Impulses from the vagina and cervix reflexly stimulate the hypothalamus to release a LH releasing factor, and this compound in turn affects the anterior lobe of the pituitary gland to secrete LH. When the level of this hormone in the blood reaches a certain level, ovulation takes place.

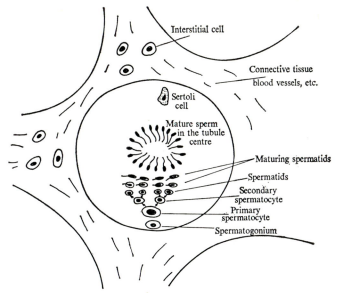

Fig.14.1. Sperm formation in the testis (from Horrobin, *Medical Physiology and Biochemistry*, by kind permission of the author and Edward Arnold, 1968).

SPERMATOGENESIS

The testis has two functions—the production of male sex hormone and the formation of spermatozoa. Each testis consists of a mass of seminiferous tubules along the walls of which the primitive germ cells are found, known as spermatogonia. The glycogen-rich Sertoli cells, whose function is believed to be the provision of sperm nutriment, are also found in the tubules. Between the tubules there is interstitial tissue containing the interstitial cells which secrete testosterone. The seminiferous tubules empty into the network of ducts known as the epididymis which in turn drains into the thick walled muscular vas deferens. The vasa deferentia empty into the urethra.

The accessory sex glands of the male are situated behind the neck of the urinary bladder and are closely related to the pelvic portion of the urethra. The openings of the prostate and seminal vesicles are close to the neck of the urinary bladder. The bulbo-urethral glands are situated more to the posterior, embedded in the skeletal muscles associated with the root of the penis or the ischial arch. When the semen passes the vas deferens and urethra the secretion from the accessory glands is added. In this way the semen is diluted and

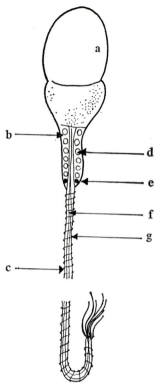

Fig.14.2. Details of mammalian spermatozoa. (a) Sperm head. (b) Mid-piece. (c) Tail. (d) Mitochondria. (e) Centriole. (f) Axial filaments. (g) Helix, which coils round the surface of tail.

nutrients and buffers are added. This creates ideal conditions for the movements of the spermatozoa and for their metabolism.

Spermatozoa

The spermatogenic process can be divided into three main stages: (1) spermatocytogenesis which is the development of the spermatogonium to primary and secondary spermatocytes, (2) meiosis in which two cell divisions occur reducing the number of chromosomes in the spermatids to half of that in spermatocytes, (3) spermiogenesis, the differentation of spermatids to spermatozoa (Fig.14.1).

Each spermatozoon consists of a head, a mid-piece, and a tail. The nucleus extending through the entire head contains the genetic material needed for fertilization of the ovum. The sperm nucleus contains half as much deoxyribonucleic acid (DNA) as the nucleus of the spermatogonium. The mid-piece contains mitochondria in which the enzyme systems associated with metabolic activity are found. They provide energy for sperm motility. The sperm tail is a very long whip-like structure. Two centrioles are located in the mid-piece. From here fibrils extend into the tail. There are two central fibrils surrounded by a ring of nine peripheral pairs of fibrils. These fibrils are presumed to facilitate the movement of the sperm (Fig. 14.2).

Semen

The semen is composed of two parts, the spermatozoa and the seminal plasma. While the spermatozoa are formed in the testis and stored in the epididymis, the seminal plasma is contributed by the secretory fluids produced in the accessory sex organs. The sperm concentration varies from species to species.

Table 14.1 Volume, sperm concentration, and pH of the ejaculate of various domestic animals

Animal	Volume (ml)	No. of spermatozoa per mm³	pH
Bull	4–8	1 000 000	6·4–7·8
Ram	0·5–2	3 000 000	5·9–7·3
Stallion	30–200	100 000	6·2–7·8
Boar	150–400	100 000	7·3–7·9

The seminal plasma is distinguished by a high content of choline, citric acid, fructose, and certain other chemical substances not found in large quantities elsewhere in the animal body. The seminal plasma acts as a buffer owing to its bicarbonate, citrate, and protein content. This of importance to protect the spermatozoa in the female genital tract where the pH is lower due to the high hydrogen concentration of the vaginal secretions.

The time that passes from first formation of the sperm to its ejaculation is usually about 50 days. This can be determined by injecting radioactive phosphate into the animal. In this way the nucleic acids in the nucleus of all cells will be marked. Since the phosphate remains in the cells, the time that passes from injection to the first appearance of radioactive spermatozoa in the ejaculate, determines the age of the cells.

Ejaculation of semen

Erection of the penis is essentially an increase in the turgidity of the organ caused by a greater inflow of blood than outflow, with resultant increase in pressure within the penis. Both dilatation of the arteries and a decrease in the venous drainage from the penis are factors in producing erection. When the penis of the horse erects a considerable increase in diameter as well as increase in length occurs because of the relatively large amounts of erectile tissue in comparison with the quantity of connective tissue. The penis of ruminants and swine erects chiefly by straightening of the sigmoid flexures. Although the turgidity increases, the length and diameter of the penis remains nearly the same as in the relaxed condition. This is due to the relatively little erectile tissue in comparison with the amount of connective tissue.

Ejaculation is a reflex emptying of the epididymis, urethra, and accessory sex glands of the male. The reflex is caused by stimulation of the glans penis, either during natural service or by the artificial vagina used for collecting semen for examination or for artificial insemination. Ejaculation can also be produced by manual massage of the accessory sex glands through the rectum or by use of an electric ejaculator.

OOGENESIS

The ovaries are the primary organs of reproduction in the female just as the testes are in the male. The ovaries may be considered to be both endocrine and cell producing in nature, since they produce hormones which are secreted directly into the blood stream and also produce ova which are expelled from the gland.

The central portion of the ovary is the most vascular part, while most of the cortex consists of dense irregular connective tissue interspersed with parenchymal epithelial cells. The outer layer of cortex is a dense connective tissue capsule.

Cords of germinal epithelial cells invade the stroma of the ovary and eventually form isolated clumps of cells known as primary follicles. One large cell in each follicle is an oocyte or ovum surrounded by a single layer of follicular cells.

Ova in primary follicles increase in size, and the follicular cells multiply into several layers forming maturing follicles. A thick membrane, the zona pellucida, appears between the ovum and the inner layer of follicular cells of the maturing follicle. As soon as a

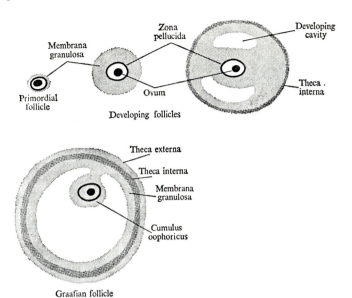

Fig.14.3. Outline of follicular development (from Horrobin, *Medical Physiology and Biochemistry*, by kind permission of the author and Edward Arnold, 1968).

fluid filled cavity appears within the mass of follicular cells the follicle may be called a Graafian follicle or vesicular follicle, and the layer of follicular cells is called the membrana granulosa. This layer is believed to be the source of oestrogen found in the follicular fluid.

Some of the membrana granulosa cells form a mound surrounding the ovum, known as the germ hill or cumulus oophoricus. The Graafian follicle continues to increase in size and pushes towards the surface of the ovary, where in some species it can be palpated via the rectum as a cyst-like bulge.

Monotocous animals (those not bearing litters) such as the horse and the cow, normally have only one offspring per gestation. At each heat period one follicle usually develops more rapidly than the others, so that when it ruptures only one ovum or egg is released and the rest of the follicles then regress and form atretic follicles.

Polytocous animals, such as pigs, which normally produce several offspring per gestation, have several follicle ruptures at the same time. The ova may all come from one ovary, or some may come from each ovary.

Immediately following ovulation the follicular cavity fills with a variable amount of blood and lymph. This is gradually replaced by the corpus luteum. The granulosa cells multiply rapidly to form the major part of the corpus luteum. These cells produce the hormone progesterone.

In contrast to the male sex cells which form four spermatozoa from each primary sex cell, the female sex cell results in only one mature ovum and three rudimentary cells. The division that produces the first rudimentary cell is meiotic in nature, that is, it is a reduction division in which the chromosome number is reduced to one half of the original number.

OESTRUS CYLCE

Domestic females come into heat at fairly regular intervals which differ rather widely between species. The interval from the beginning of one heat period to the beginning of the next is called the oestrus cycle. It is controlled directly by hormones from the ovary and indirectly by hormones from the anterior lobe of the pituitary gland. The oestrus cycle is divided into several well-marked phases called proestrus, oestrus, metoestrus, and dioestrus. Aneostrus is a period of total sexual quiescence between oestrus cycles.

Proestrus

Under stimulation of FSH from the anterior lobe of the pituitary gland, the ovary produces increasing quantities of oestrogen. It is during this phase that the ovarian follicle, with its enclosed ovum, increases in size primarily by increasing the volume of follicular

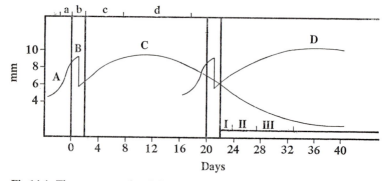

Fig.14.4. The oestrus cycle of the sow. The ordinate is the diameter of follicle and corpus luteum. (A) Growth of follicle. (B) Ovulation. (C) Corpus luteum in non-pregnant sow. (D) Corpus luteum in pregnant sow. (a) Proestrus. (b) Estrus. (c) Metoestrus. (d) Dioestrus. (I) Eggs in Fallopian tube. (II) Eggs in uterus. (III) Implantation begins.

fluid. Oestrogen absorbed from the follicles into the blood stream stimulates the vascularity and cell growth of the uterus and vagina in preparation for oestrus and subsequent pregnancy.

Oestrus

Oestrus is the period of sexual receptivity in the female, which is determined largely by the level of circulating oestrogen. During or shortly after this period ovulation occurs, and the corpus luteum begins to form at the time LH from the anterior lobe of the pituitary gland increases and FSH decreases. Just before ovulation the follicle is large and turgid, and the enclosed ovum undergoes maturation changes. Oestrus terminates about the time that rupture of the ovarian follicle occurs. At this point the ovum is expelled from the follicle to pass into the upper part of the Fallopian tube.

Metoestrus

Metoestrus is the post-ovulatory phase during which the corpus luteum develops. The length of metoestrus may depend on the length of time for which LH is secreted. During this period there is a decrease in oestrogen and an increase in progesterone formed by the ovary. The progesterone prevents further development of follicles and hence the occurrence of further oestrous periods. Progesterone is necessary for proper implantation of the fertilized ovum in the uterus, for nourishment of the developing embryo, and for development of the alveoli of the mammary gland.

Dioestrus

Dioestrus is a relatively short period between oestrous cycles in polyoestrous animals when there is a mature corpus luteum. Anoestrus is a longer period between breeding seasons.

FERTILIZATION

In general ovulation occurs near the end of oestrus or shortly after oestrus has terminated. At ovulation the eggs are liberated onto the surface of the ovary, and from there into the infundibulum, which is the funnel shaped ovarian end of the Fallopian tube. The site of fertilization is the ampulla of the Fallopian tube. The eggs of domestic animals remain fully viable for 12–24 hours after ovulation. Loss of viability is not sudden: ageing eggs may be able to undergo apparently normal fertilization, but will give rise to embryos that die before birth. With further deterioration, fertilization becomes abnormal or fails altogether.

At coitus semen is passed into the female reproductive tract. The volume of the ejaculate varies (see Table 14.1). In the mare the semen is projected into the cranial end of the vagina and through the relaxed cervical canal into the uterus. In the pig the voluminous ejaculate is slowly propelled through vagina and cervix into the uterus during the prolonged coitus. In cattle and sheep the volume of the ejaculate is small, and is deposited in the cranial end of the vagina.

The spermatozoa move through the female genital tract only slightly by their own motility and mostly because of contractions of the uterine wall. The transport of spermatozoa to the ampulla of the Fallopian tube is remarkably rapid: periods of 15 minutes or less have been reported for the cow. Dead spermatozoa are transported as fast as living ones, which serves to emphasize the small contribution of the cells' own motility.

Normally coitus takes place early in the heat period so that the spermatozoa will reach the site of fertilization several hours before the eggs. With artificial insemination, however, unless due care is taken, there is a risk that the natural time relations will be disturbed and the chance of fertilization thus reduced.

The total number of spermatozoa in a single ejaculate is approximately 6000×10^6 in the stallion, 3000×10^6 in the bull, 800×10^6 in the ram, and $20\,000 \times 10^6$ in the boar. These are enormous numbers and represent in each instance very many more spermatozoa than are necessary for normal fertility. If, for example, an average bull ejaculate is suitably diluted and used for artificial insemination of about 500 cows, the great majority of them are likely to become pregnant. The number of spermatozoa that reaches the Fallopian tubes is much reduced, in the order of thousands. In general the spermatozoa are incapable of retaining full viability and fertility in the female genital tract for more than 24 hours. The arrival of the spermatozoa at the site of fertilization before the eggs suggests that spermatozoa are not capable of participating in fertilization immediately upon entering the female tract, but must reside there for a period to develop this capacity.

The meeting of eggs and spermatozoa is the resultant of several interacting influences and conditions. Basically they depend upon the speed of movement of the spermatozoa, the concentration of spermatozoa around the eggs, and the surface area of the eggs.

Concentration of spermatozoa can probably be taken as chief variable. The significance of a small number of spermatozoa at the site of fertilization deserves emphasis. The participation of more than one spermatozoa in fertilization is a pathological occurrence and almost certainly leads to early death of the embryo. As eggs themselves have imperfect protection against the penetration of more than one spermatozoa, it is important that the chances of fertilization should not surpass a certain upper limit. It is of equal importance, of course, that they should not fall below a certain limit, if fertility is to be maintained. The control of the transport of spermatozoa is, therefore, important in order that the number reaching the site of fertilization be sufficient to provide good chances of fertilization for all eggs, without being so large as to cause serious risk of polyspermi.

Fertilization involves the penetration of the spermatozoa into the egg, the formation of a spermatozoa pronucleus and an egg pronucleus, the growth of these pronuclei, the replacement of the pronuclei by chromosome groups, and finally the union of the two chromosome groups. The essential feature of fertilization lies in the mingling of paternal and maternal chromosomes. By this act chromosomes from two different sources are brought together to constitute the genetic material of the new individual and the diploid chromosome number is restored.

DEVELOPMENT OF THE FOETUS

The conclusion of fertilization marks the genesis of the zygote or early embryo. Initially the main feature of development is a special form of cell division known as cleavage during which the protoplasmatic mass of the embryo is progressively divided until it composes a large number of cells. Cleavage involves no gain, rather some loss of total protoplasmatic matter. It continues until the cells constituting the embryo are of the size that is normal for the tissues of the animal concerned. Cleavage then ceases, but cell division continues associated with increase in total mass, that is to say with the growth of the embryo.

After fertilization the embryo passes down the Fallopian tube and in a few days enters the uterus. Eventually the embryo undergoes implantation in the uterus, a process involving the formation of a placenta to which both embryonic and maternal tissues contribute. The nutritive requirements of the embryo are met initially by the yolk material that it carries, by substances in the secretion of the Fallopian tube, and later by the products of the uterine glands. Ultimately, the embryo is maintained through the medium of the placenta.

The placenta consists of an arrangement of membranes such that nutrients from the dam can reach the foetus and waste products from the foetus can be excreted by the dam. The placenta, or foetal membranes, include the chorion, allantois, amnion, and the remaining part of the yolk sac.

Table 14.2 The reproductive cycle in domestic animals

Species	Nature of cycles	Duration of cycles (days)		Duration of oestrus		Time of ovulation	Duration of pregnancy (days)		Age of puberty
		Average	Variation	Average	Variation		Average	Variation	
Mare	Polyoestrus (seasonal; in spring)	22	16–30	6 days	2–11 days	1–2 days before end of oestrus	336	329–346	One year
Ass	Polyoestrus (seasonal; in spring)	23	13–31	6 days	2–14 days	Last third of oestrus	365	—	One year
Cow	Polyoestrus (all year)	21	18–24	16 hours	8–30 hours	10 hours after end of oestrus	282	274–291	12–15 months
Ewe	Polyoestrus (seasonal; in autumn. More extensive in some breeds)	16½	14–20	35 hours	1–3 days	At end of oestrus	150	140–160	One year
Goat	Polyoestrus (seasonal; in autumn)	About 21	15–24	2½ days	2–3 days	Toward end of oestrus	151	140–160	One year
Sow	Polyoestrus (all year)	21	18–24	2–3 days	1–5 days	Toward end of oestrus	113	110–116	3–5 months
Rabbit	Polyoestrus (all year, except tendency toward anoestrum in summer)	—	—	One month	?	Induced, 10½ hours after coitus	31	30–32	About 6 months

The nature of the cycles for animals in temperate zones are shown in brackets

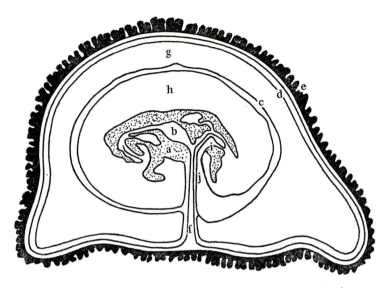

Fig.14.5. Foetus of a horse within the placenta. (a) Foetus. (b) Digestive tract.
(c) Amnion. (d) Allantois. (e) Chorion. (f) Yolk sac. (g) Allantois sac. (h) Amnion
sac. (i) Bladder. (j) Urachus.

The chorion, the outer membrane, is in contact with the uterus.
The amnion is the inner membrane, closest to the foetus. The
allantoic sac is a space formed by the two layers of allantois, located
between amnion and chorion. This sac is continuous with the
anterior extremity of the bladder by way of the urachus via the
umbilical cord. The outer layer of allantois is fused to the chorion by
connective tissue, and the inner layer of allantois is fused to the
amnion. The amnionic sac surrounds the foetus (Fig.14.5).

Branches of the umbilical arteries and veins are located in the
connective tissues between the allantois and chorion. The umbilical
arteries and their branches carry unoxygenated blood from the
foetus to the placenta, and the umbilical veins carry oxygenated
blood from the placenta to the foetus. As a general principle blood
from the foetus never mixes with blood from the dam. However, the
two circulations are close enough at the junction of chorion and
endometrium for oxygen and nutrients to pass from the maternal to
the foetal blood, and for waste products to pass in the opposite
direction. The exact relationship between the blood vessels of the
foetus and the dam depends on the species and the type of placenta
involved.

The haemochorial type of placenta is found in humans and some types of rodents. Here the chorion of the foetal placenta, including the foetal vessels, is invaginated into pools of maternal blood. Three layers separate the blood of the foetus from that of the mother, the endothelium of the chorion capillary, the connective tissue, and the trophoblast layer of the chorion.

The endotheliochorial type of placenta is found in carnivorous animals. Here the chorion of the foetal placenta is in contact with the endothelium of the blood vessels of the dam. Four layers separate the foetus and the dam, the endothelium, connective tissue, and trophoblast layer of the chorion and the endothelium of the maternal capillaries.

The epitheliochorial placenta is found in horses, pigs and ruminants. Here chorionic villi which cover much of the foetal placenta project into crypts scattered over the entire endometrium of the uterus. The chorion of the foetal placenta is in contact with the epithelium of the endometrium of the uterus. The blood of the foetus is separated from that of the dam by six layers of tissue, the endothelium, the connective tissue, and the trophoblast layer of the chorion and the epithelium, the connective tissue, and the endothelium of the endometrium.

PREGNANCY DIAGNOSIS

The knowledge of whether a breeding female is pregnant or not is of considerable importance to a livestock breeder. There are a number of criteria which may be used to help determine if a female is pregnant and how long she has been pregnant: (1) absence of oestrus. If accurate records of oestrus periods and breeding dates are kept, the earliest indication of pregnancy is failure to come into heat in the next expected period. Such an absence of oestrus, however, is not absolute proof of pregnancy; (2) change of contour of abdomen. As pregnancy advances in any female a definite dropping of the abdominal wall occurs as well as a widening of the abdomen; (3) palpation per rectum. Pregnancy can be diagnosed with a high degree of accuracy by rectal palpation in cattle and horses. The diagnosis of pregnancy and the estimation of stage of pregnancy are based upon knowledge of the rate of development of the foetus and changes in the genitalia and associated structures of the dam; (4) chemical and biological tests based upon the presence of gonadotrophins or oestrogens in blood or urine are used in the mare and human.

NOURISHMENT OF THE FOETUS

In the early stages of foetal life the new organism is nourished by secretions from the uterine glands. These secretions contain 10–12 per cent protein, 1–2 per cent lipid, and small amounts of carbohydrate and minerals.

When the placenta is developed nutrients can pass from the maternal blood to the foetal blood, and waste products can pass in the opposite direction. The following factors are of importance in the transfer of nutrients from the maternal to the foetal blood; (1) the concentration of oxygen and nutrients in the maternal blood. During pregnancy the amount of amino acids, glucose, iron, and copper increases in the dam; (2) the flow-rate of blood in the uterus. The volume of blood that passes the uterus is increased by 30–40 per cent during pregnancy; (3) the area of contact between the foetal and maternal placenta. This area decreases with the number of foetuses in the uterus.

Proteins and amino acids

In animals with a thin placenta barrier the blood plasma of the foetus will have the same composition as that of the dam, whereas in animals with a thick placenta like horses, pigs, and ruminants, they differ considerably. The foetal blood in these animals contains no gamma-globulin, and therefore the new born animals lack antibodies. In such animals the antibodies are received with the colostrum.

In animals with a thin placental barrier both amino acids and intact protein are transferred across the placenta, whereas in animals with a thick barrier only amino acids are transported. The placenta transport of amino acids is an active energy requiring process, since the foetal blood has a higher amino acid concentration than the maternal blood and a different composition.

Carbohydrates

In animals with a thin placental barrier the blood glucose concentration of the foetal blood is identical to that of the maternal blood, whereas in animals with a thick placenta the foetal blood glucose concentration is higher than the maternal. This indicates that the latter type of placenta transports glucose by an active mechanism.

Lipids

The concentration of lipids in the foetal blood is lower than in the maternal blood, and the composition differs in that the foetal blood contains relatively more unsaturated fatty acids. This indicates that the lipids are broken down in the placenta cells, and the components transferred to the foetal blood or utilized in resynthesis of lipids that are transferred to the foetus.

Inorganic compounds

Sodium, potassium, and chloride pass the placenta by passive diffusion and are found in the same concentrations as in foetal and maternal blood. Calcium and phosphate are absorbed by an active process and occur in higher concentrations in foetal than in maternal blood.

The actual mechanism for iron transport across the placental barrier is unknown, but it seems to be regulated by the foetal requirements rather than by the concentration of iron in the maternal blood.

Vitamins

The transport mechanisms for vitamins are unknown. The fat soluble vitamins are found in lower concentrations, whereas the water soluble vitamins are found in higher concentrations in the foetal blood than in the maternal blood.

Water

The transport of water from maternal to foetal blood is under influence of hydrostatic, osmotic, and colloid osmotic forces on both sides of the placental barrier.

Oxygen and carbon dioxide

Both oxygen and carbon dioxide move across the placenta in accordance with concentration gradients. The partial pressure of oxygen is higher in maternal than in foetal blood and so oxygen moves from mother to foetus. The partial pressure of carbon dioxide, on the other hand, is higher in the foetus and so carbon dioxide moves from foetus to mother.

The transfer of oxygen is facilitated by the fact that the foetus has a different type of haemoglobin (known appropriately as foetal haemoglobin) from that in the adult animal. Foetal haemoglobin

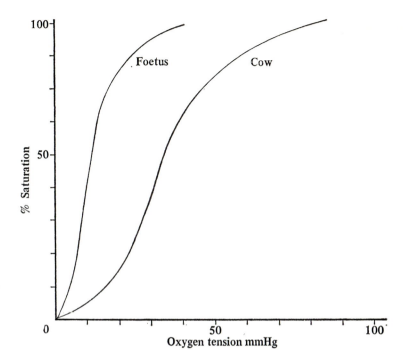

Fig.14.6. Oxygen dissociation curves for maternal and foetal blood in cattle.

has a much higher affinity for oxygen and so can become saturated at lower partial pressures as shown in Fig.14.6. Soon after birth the production of foetal haemoglobin stops and normal adult haemoglobin is made instead.

ENDOCRINE MECHANISM DURING PREGNANCY

During pregnancy the corpus luteum persists and continues producing progesterone. The persistence of the corpus luteum is caused by stimulation of LH produced by the anterior lobe of the pituitary gland and by a similar hormone produced by the placenta. In some animals progesterone is produced by the placenta in the later stages of pregnancy. In such animals removal of the corpus luteum will cause abortion in the first period of pregnancy, but not usually in the later stages.

The production of progesterone, whether produced by the corpus luteum or the placenta, will decline toward the end of pregnancy and

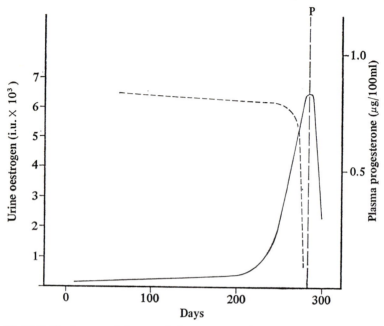

Fig.14.7. The hormonal changes during pregnancy in a cow. P = parturition.
—Oestrogen concentration in urine. ....Progesterone concentration in plasma.

the placental production of oestrogens will increase. In the period of high progesterone production the motility of the uterus is very weak, because progesterone inhibits the action of oxytocin on the myometrium. The decrease in progesterone and increase in oestrogen production changes the oxytocin susceptibility of the myometrium and uterine contractions begin to occur. Finally the contractions of the uterine wall become very forceful, the animal is in labour (Fig. 14.7).

In the last part of pregnancy a non-steroid hormone is formed by the ovaries, the endometrium, and the placenta. This hormone causes relaxation of the cervix muscles and of the pelvic ligaments.

Parturition

The act of giving birth marks the termination of pregnancy. Parturition is divided into three stages. The first stage consists of uterine contractions which gradually force the fluid filled foetal membranes against the uterine side of the cervix, causing it to dilate. This stage lasts 2–6 hours in the cow and ewe, 1–4 hours in the mare, and 2–12 hours in the sow. In the second stage actual delivery of the foetus occurs. Passage of parts of the foetus through the cervix into the vagina along with rupture of the foetal membranes initiates contraction of the abdominal muscle. The continuation of uterine and abdominal contractions forces the foetus through the birth canal. The third stage of parturition consists of delivery of the placenta, which normally follows the foetus almost immediately.

The initiation of parturition is not well understood but the latest evidence indicates that it is started off by a surge of cortisol production by the foetal adrenal glands.

15

Lactation

MILK SECRETION

Mammary growth and lactation represent important phases of the reproduction cycle of mammals. Milk provides an essential and highly digestible form of nutrient for the young during the critical period after birth. The same hormones which control growth and function of the uterus also control growth and function of the mammary glands. Extensive growth does not usually begin until gestation and is largely completed by the end of the first two thirds of pregnancy. After the onset of lactation at parturition, milk production rises for a relatively brief period and then gradually declines, and the lobuloalveolar system undergoes involution. These events are repeated after the next cycle of fertilization and pregnancy.

It has been shown that ovarian hormones are largely responsible for mammary growth, with oestrogens stimulating growth of ducts and progesterone stimulating alveolar growth. However, removal of the pituitary gland reduces the effect of the ovarian hormones on development of the mammary glands. Hormones responsible for this pituitary effect are thyrotrophic hormone, growth hormone, ACTH, and prolactin.

Initiation of lactation

Injection of prolactin into an animal with fully developed mammary glands causes secretion of milk. The balance of oestrogen and progesterone maintained by the placenta during pregnancy inhibits either the release or the action of prolactin. Following parturition the inhibition by the placental hormones is removed and prolactin initiates milk secretion. Retention of the placenta after parturition causes inhibition of milk secretion in cows. Suckling stimulates the production of prolactin from the pituitary gland.

Milk is formed in the epithelial cells of the alveoli of the mammary glands. When filled with milk each alveolus is about 0·2 mm in diameter. The alveoli are grouped together in structures known as lobules which are surrounded by connective tissue. Each lobule is approximately one cubic millimetre in volume. The lobules are in turn grouped to form larger units called lobes which are also surrounded by layers of connective tissue.

The alveoli discharge their milk into small ducts. These join together to give larger ducts which eventually empty into the spaces (cisternae) above the teat. The opening in the teat is known as the streak canal. In cattle the primary structure responsible for retention of milk is a sphincter muscle which surrounds the streak canal. In sheep the closure of the canal is due to elastic connective tissue rather than to circular smooth muscle fibres forming a sphincter. In pigs each teat has two streak canals which are normally kept closed by longitudinal folds of mucosa; only a few muscle fibres are found.

Regulation of milk secretion

If the secretion present in the ducts and alveoli at the time of parturition is removed, either by the young suckling or by milking, the production of milk will start and continue for a period, known as the lactation period. In the first part of this period the daily secretion increases, after which it slowly declines. Milk production in sows is highest approximately 2 weeks after parturition, whereas in cows the highest daily production is reached 3–6 weeks after parturition (Fig.15.1).

In the course of the first lactation period the capacity of the mammary gland increases, and maximal milk production in cattle is reached in the 6th or 7th lactation period.

The duration of the lactation period and the daily milk production varies among races and individuals. Generally speaking, a normal milking cow, weighing 500–600 kg, should be able to produce an average of 20–30 kg of milk daily in the first two months of the lactation period. In goats the maximum production is approximately 2–3 kg, and in sows the maximum daily milk production is 8–11 kg.

If the animal becomes pregnant during the lactation period the daily milk production will fall. In cows this inhibition begins about 3 months after conception, and is caused by the production of hormones by the corpus luteum and placenta. If the cow does not become pregnant during the lactation period, milk production will

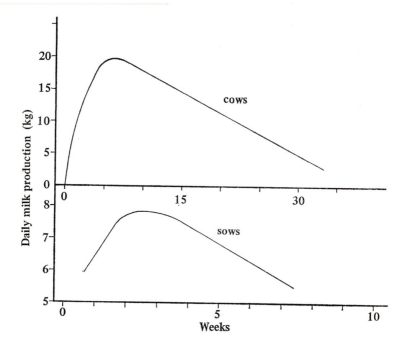

Fig.15.1. The lactation curves for cows and sows.

decrease, but at a slower rate. This reduction in milk production is caused by the hormones produced by the ovaries. Removal of the ovaries in the early stage of lactation will cause the milk production to continue for a prolonged period of time.

Secretion of milk is a continuous process, although it does not occur at a constant rate. Immediately following milking the pressure in the ducts and alveoli is at its lowest, and secretion occurs at its maximum rate. In the hours following milking the pressure increases owing to accumulation of milk in the gland, and secretion gradually decreases. When the pressure in the mammary gland reaches approximately 40 mmHg, secretion ceases due to closure of the capillaries and a fall in the blood flow (Fig.15.2).

Milk ejection

As a result of secretion, milk will accumulate in the alveoli and ducts. This causes a rise in tension of the myoepithelial cells of the mammary gland. This increased tension, however, causes no contraction of the myoepithelial cells.

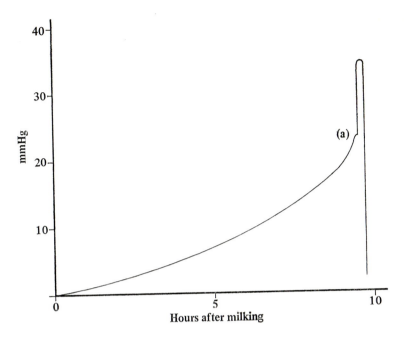

Fig.15.2. Pressure in the mammary ducts of a cow before and after milk let down (a).

Contraction of the cells and consequent ejection of the milk only occurs following stimulation of the teats, either by the young suckling or by washing the teats with a damp cloth. This suckling or milk let-down reflex is neurohormonal and involves afferent neurons from the skin of the teats to the posterior lobe of the pituitary gland. The stimulus causes release of the hormone oxytocin, which reaches the mammary gland via the blood and causes the myoepithelial cells to contract (Figs.15.2 and 15.3).

In cattle the pressure increase in the mammary gland begins 30–40 seconds after the stimulation of the teats and lasts for 4–6 minutes. Besides the contraction of the myoepithelial cells, oxytocin also causes a dilatation of the sphincter muscles closing the teat canal.

The milk ejection reflex can be conditioned to stimuli associated with milking routine, such as feeding, noise of buckets, and washing of the udder. It can also be inhibited by emotional disturbance such as dogs barking, loud unfamiliar noises, and painful treatment. It is uncertain whether this is due to decreased oxytocin output, or to reduced mammary blood flow as a result of activation of the sympathetic nervous system by adrenalin.

Failure to get adequate milk ejection due to constriction of the teat canal occurs in cows. Because of excessive retention of milk in the udder, the lactation period of such an animal may be shortened. Since the condition is genetic such animals should be excluded from breeding.

COMPOSITION AND SYNTHESIS OF MILK

Colostrum

The first milk secreted after parturition, known as colostrum, is rich in minerals, vitamins, and proteins. In mares, cows, and sows colostrum contains up to 25 per cent proteins, the majority of which are gamma-globulins. Colostrum is of great importance to the new-born animal, especially in species with a thick placental barrier, e.g. calves, foals, and pigs. These animals are born without antibody-containing gamma-globulins. In the first days after birth the intestinal epithelium is permeable to intact protein molecules, and the young animal obtains passive immunity until it can develop its own antibodies.

Normal milk

Normal milk is a suspension of fat droplets in the milk plasma. The milk plasma is a colloid and crystalloid solution of protein, lactose, and minerals (Table 15.1). The composition of milk varies between species, and within species there are racial and individual differences. Besides these genetic differences, the composition of milk may be altered by external factors such as composition of feed and number of daily milkings.

Milk fat is present as droplets ranging from 3–5 μ in diameter in cows. Milk fat is mainly composed of triglycerides. The fatty acids are mainly short-chain fatty acids ranging from 4–12 carbon atoms each. These short-chain fatty acids are not generally found in the storage fats of animals. Milk fat may be synthesized either by breaking down long-chain fatty acids found in the circulating blood or by synthesis from other substances.

Non-ruminants appear to use glucose, and ruminants use acetate for synthesis of milk fat. The short-chain fatty acids, the length of palmitic acid or shorter in cows' milk, are formed from acetate, whereas the long-chain fatty acids are probably formed from blood glycerides.

Milk protein mainly consists of casein, a phosphoprotein that is found only in milk. Small amounts of lactoalbumin and lacto-globulin are also present in milk. Milk proteins may be synthesized by uniting amino acids, by degradation of plasma proteins, by rearrangements of peptide chains in plasma proteins, or by a combination of all three methods. Blood passing through the udder of a lactating cow decreases in amino acid content, but the quantity of amino acids taken up does not appear sufficient to account for the formation of total milk protein.

Table 15.1 The composition of milk from domestic animals

Animal	Dry matter	Total protein	Casein	Fat	Lactose	Minerals	kcal per 100 g	Doubling of birth weight (days)
		Content (percentage by weight)						
Cow	12·8	3·5	2·8	3·8	4·8	0·7	79	45
Goat	12·8	3·7	2·9	4·1	4·2	0·8	80	20
Ewe	16·8	5·4	4·3	6·2	4·3	0·9	108	13
Mare	10·7	2·5	1·6	1·6	6·1	0·5	55	60
Sow	20·4	6·3	4·4	7·7	5·6	0·8	133	16

The udder appears to take up specific amino acids in approximately the same proportion as they exist in casein. All of the casein may be formed from amino acids, the other proteins may be derived, at least in part, from peptide portions of plasma proteins.

Lactose is a disaccharide normally found only in the mammary gland and in milk. Glucose is the major substance used by the mammary gland to form lactose, since the venous blood leaving the udder contains less glucose than the arterial blood entering it. Experimentally mammary gland tissue homogenates have produced lactose with glucose as the only substrate.

The amounts of water soluble vitamins vary considerably between species, but are independent of the feeding. The amounts of fat soluble vitamins on the other hand depends on the amount eaten. The amounts of minerals and vitamins in the milk of various animals are shown in Table 15.2.

Table 15.2 The concentration of minerals and vitamins in the milk of domestic animals (per 100 ml) (from Moustgaard).

	Cow		Ewe	Goat	Mare		Sow
	Colostrum	Milk	Milk	Milk	Milk	Colostrum	Milk
Sodium (mg)	60	50	70	—	60	75	30
Potassium (mg)	150	150	90	—	120	125	90
Calcium (mg)	170	120	160	140	100	50	240
Magnesium (mg)	15	10	20	15	10	—	—
Phosphorus (mg)	—	90	150	120	60	80	150
Iron (μg)	200	50	—	—	—	300	100
Copper (μg)	50	20	—	—	—	—	50
Vit. A (i.u.)	700	120	150	120	50	200	120
Vit. D (i.u.)	4	3	3	2	—	—	4
Vit. E (mg)	2	0·4	—	—	—	—	—
Thiamin (μg)	60	30	70	50	30	100	65
Riboflavin (μg)	500	170	500	120	20	135	200
Niacin (μg)	100	100	500	200	50	165	400
Pantothenic acid (μg)	220	300	350	350	500	130	500
Vit. B_6 (μg)	50	50	—	—	30	10	40
Vit. B_{12} (μg)	1·0	0·4	0·3	0·1	0·3	0·6	0·2
Ascorbic acid (mg)	2·5	2	3	2	10	30	18

FACTORS INFLUENCING MILK PRODUCTION

Under optimal conditions the synthesis of milk is determined by the number of secreting cells, and by the capacity of the cells. The number of cells is determined by genetic factors, whereas the secretory capacity is influenced by external factors such as feeding and climatic conditions.

During a single lactation period a milking cow secretes several times the amount of protein, fat, and minerals present in its own body. At the same time the cow must meet the demands for development of the foetus. Lack of sufficient feed will cause inhibition of milk secretion due to decreased amounts of necessary compounds for milk synthesis in the blood. The function of the secretory cells may also be inhibited due to lack of essential nutritional factors, and the endocrine system may be disturbed by insufficiency in specific factors.

Climate

Changes in the surrounding temperatures outside the thermoneutral zone lead to decreases or increases of energy metabolism, caused by a change in the endocrine balance. The milk fat content of European cattle races tends to fall when the air temperature reaches 21–22 °C. At higher temperatures (24–25 °C) the amount of milk produced tends to decrease.

16

Heat production and temperature regulation

ENERGY METABOLISM

In a 10 hour period a guinea pig produces about the same amount of heat as that produced by burning 3·3 g of carbon, and the carbon dioxide produced in the 10 hour period is the same as that produced by burning the 3·3 g of carbon. It can also be demonstrated that there is the same relationship between oxygen consumption and heat production, regardless of whether carbon is burned inside the body or outside it.

Direct calorimetry

The heat produced by an animal can be measured in an ice calorimeter. This consists of a chamber for the animal, surrounded by another chamber filled with ice. The amount of heat produced by the animal is determined by measuring the amount of ice melted during a given period, and by multiplying the volume of water by the latent heat of ice, which is 79 cal/g.

Indirect calorimetry

Metabolism of 1 g of fat yields 9·3 cal, and 1 g of carbohydrate yields 4·1 cal. Since they are both completely oxidized to carbon dioxide and water, the same values would be obtained by burning 1 g of fat or 1 g of carbohydrate outside the body. Protein yields 5·3 cal when burned outside the body, but only 4·1 when metabolized. This difference in heat production is due to the excretion of nitrogenous waste products from protein metabolism. The difference practically disappears when the heat equivalent of the urine and faeces is added to the metabolic figure for protein.

The production of heat per litre of oxygen consumed depends on what compounds are metabolized. Determination of this production, therefore, demands a determination of the amounts of protein, fat, and carbohydrates metabolized in the experimental period. This determination is based upon the excretion of nitrogen in the urine and the amount of oxygen consumed and carbon dioxide excreted. The ratio, carbon dioxide expired divided by oxygen inspired $\dfrac{CO_2}{O_2}$ is known as the respiratory quotient. The respiratory quotient of carbohydrate is 1·0, since one molecule of carbon dioxide is produced for each molecule of oxygen used. Fats contain relatively less oxygen than carbohydrates, so more molecules of oxygen are required than molecules of carbon dioxide produced. Some of the oxygen is used to oxidize a portion of the hydrogen to water. This gives a respiratory quotient of 0·7. Proteins give a respiratory quotient of 0·8.

The amount of protein metabolized is calculated from the excretion of nitrogen in the urine (urine-nitrogen × 6·25). The amount of oxygen consumed and carbon dioxide excreted due to protein metabolism, can then be calculated (see Table 16.1), and subtracted from the total oxygen consumption and carbon dioxide excretion. The respiratory quotient of metabolized nitrogen free compounds

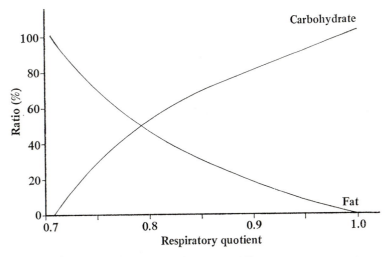

Fig.16.1. The ratio of fat and carbohydrate at different respiratory quotients (see text).

can then be found, and based on this value the ratio of carbo-hydrate to fat (Fig.16.1) can be calculated.

Table 16.1 Heat production, oxygen consumption, and carbon dioxide production of metabolism

	Heat production		Litre O_2 used per gram	Litre CO_2 produced per gram	Respiratory quotient
	Total kcal/g	In organism kcal/g			
Carbohydrate	4·2	4·2	0·83	0·83	1·00
Fat	9·5	9·5	2·02	1·43	0·71
Protein	5·7	4·5	0·97	0·78	0·81

Basal metabolism

Basal metabolism refers to the amount of heat produced by an animal at complete rest 12–14 hours after eating. It may be regarded as the lowest possible heat production. The release of energy is a result of catabolism of the animal's own tissue.

Basal metabolism depends on the surface area of the body and on the weight of the animal. Approximate basal metabolism values per 24 hours are: cattle (500 kg; 6·7 m²) 6600 kcal, pigs (100 kg; 2·2 m²) 2000 kcal, sheep (40 kg; 1·2 m²) 1000 kcal.

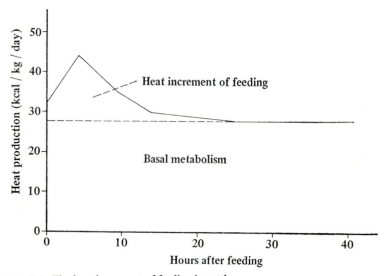

Fig.16.2. The heat increment of feeding in cattle.

When an animal eats, an immediate rise in heat production, known as heat increment of feeding, is recorded (Fig.16.2). The extent of this increase in metabolism rate depends on the amount of feed and its composition.

TEMPERATURE REGULATION

Based upon the relationship between their body temperature and the surrounding temperature, animals can be divided into two groups, the cold blooded or poikilothermic and the warm blooded or homeothermic animals. The cold blooded animals change their body temperature according to the surrounding temperature, whereas the warm blooded animals are able to regulate their heat production and heat loss in such a way that the body temperature is kept constant in spite of considerable changes in the surrounding temperatures.

Table 16.2 Rectal temperature of domestic animals in °C

Animal	Rectal temperature
Horse	37·5–38·0
Foal	38·0–39·0
Cattle	38·0–39·0
Calf	39·0–40·0
Sheep	39·0–40·0
Goat	39·0–40·0
Pig	38·5–39·5

The body temperature measured in the rectum varies between species. As a general rule the temperature is slightly higher in young animals than in older (Table 16.2).

An increase in body temperature is known as fever. This condition is initiated by pyrogens, which are compounds that can be isolated from bacteria and may also be released by granulocytes. The pyrogens act directly on the hypothalamus. The fever is initiated by a cutting down of heat loss and perhaps an increase in heat production by shivering. Once the steady state is reached, regulation operates as before but around the new level. When the increased body temperature returns to normal, large amounts of heat must be released. A rise in body temperature of 3 °C in a cow weighing 500 kg, is equivalent to $500 \times 3 \times 0·83 = 1245$ kcal. (Specific heat of the body = 0·83.) This amount represents approximately one fifth of the basal metabolism, and the animal must get rid of it.

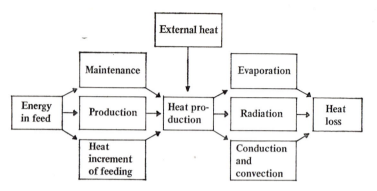

Fig. 16.3 Principal methods by which heat is produced and lost.

Heat balance

The maintenance of a constant body temperature requires that the animal is in thermal equilibrium. This means that heat production is equal to heat loss. To maintain thermal equilibrium the animal may alter either the heat production or the heat loss, the former by a change in the metabolic rate, the latter by changing the heat loss from the body surface or the respiratory tract.

Heat loss depends to a large extent on the skin temperature. By means of the arterio-venous anastomoses blood is shunted into or out of the superficial capillaries according to the demand for loss or preservation of heat in the body.

Heat transfer between the body and the environment occurs by the methods of conduction, convection, radiation, and evaporation. Conduction is heat exchange between two media in close contact. An animal can in this way lose heat to the ground when lying down. Convection is heat transfer to moving air or water. Radiation is transfer of heat from one body to another without changing the air temperature. Radiation depends only on the difference in temperature between the two objects, not on the air temperature. An example of this type of heat transfer is solar radiation. Evaporation of water releases 0·58 kcal per gram. The amount of heat lost in this way depends upon the relative humidity of the air. If the relative humidity approaches 100 per cent no evaporation can take place. Evaporative heat loss can be increased by sweating, licking or panting. The ability to secrete sweat differs with species. A human can loose 1·8–2·0 litres of water per hour per m² body surface, which equals a heat loss of 1000 kcal, or 20 times the basal metabolic rate at heat production. In cattle the maximal evaporation from the skin is 160 ml per m² per hour, equal to approximately 90 kcal, or twice the basal metabolic heat production. In small ruminants a relatively large proportion of the evaporative heat loss results from panting, and only a minor part from sweating. In large ruminants the opposite situation exists.

Control mechanisms

The reflex and semireflex thermoregulatory responses include autonomic, somatic, endocrine, and behavioural changes. One group of responses increases heat loss and decreases heat production, the other decreases heat loss and increases heat production.

If an animal is exposed to cold, it will try to increase its heat production by increased voluntary and involuntary activity (shivering), by increasing its feed uptake, and by increased secretion of adrenalin. Prolonged exposure to cold causes increased production of thyroid hormone, and therefore a higher basal metabolism. The animal exposed to cold further tries to decrease its heat loss by cutaneous vasoconstriction and erection of hair. When the surrounding temperature falls below a certain level, the animal can no longer compensate, and the body temperature falls.

Exposed to heat the animal increases its heat loss by cutaneous vasodilatation, sweating, and increased respiration. It further decreases its heat production by a low feed intake and by becoming lethargic. A prolonged heat stress causes decreased thyroid gland function and thus a lower basal metabolism. When the surrounding temperature reaches a certain level the animal can no longer adjust, and the body temperature rises.

IMPORTANCE OF ENVIRONMENT ON ANIMAL PRODUCTION

The interval between the lowest and highest readily tolerated temperatures, known as the thermoneutral zone, differs in various species and races. In the sheep the rectal temperature begins to rise above normal at an external temperature of 32 °C and panting starts at a rectal temperature of 41 °C. When the humidity is less than 65 per cent the sheep can tolerate for hours an air temperature of 43 °C. Both sweating and panting are of importance for temperature regulation in this animal and both become much less effective methods of heat loss when the humidity is high.

Sweating is very important in cattle and the sweat gland activity rises in response to a rise in external temperature and to direct solar radiation. In North European cattle races the optimal temperature is between 10 and 20 °C. Below 10 °C the skin temperature falls and metabolism increases. Prolonged exposure causes growth of hair. The heat loss is mainly due to convection and radiation. Above 20 °C the skin temperature rises and evaporation from the skin increases. At 25 °C the heat loss from evaporation exceeds that from convection and radiation. At temperatures above 25 °C the respiration rate increases. At this temperature the appetite is affected and consequently milk production falls. Air temperatures above 30–35 °C cause increases in rectal temperature. Exposed to such a heat stress over a length of time the animal adjusts by lowering the function of the thyroid gland. Under such conditions the animal is unable to maintain a high milk production as the secretory function of the mammary gland is under the influence of thyroxine. In very hot and humid climates the productivity of dairy cows can be increased considerably by keeping animals in shade, and by showering them with water several times daily. The heat tolerance varies between cattle races. Zebu cattle and related races such as the Jersey cattle have a thermoneutral zone 5–7 °C above that of the North European races.

The rectal temperature of the pig begins to rise at an air temperature of between 30 and 32 °C. If the humidity is high, the pig cannot tolerate prolonged exposure to a temperature of 35 °C. At 40 °C the pig is unable to stand an atmosphere of high humidity.

SUGGESTED READING

Cutherbertson, D. C. (editor). The Science of Nutrition of Farm Livestock. International Encyclopaedia of Food and Nutrition, Vol. 17, chapters 3, 4, 5, 11.

Frandson, R. D. Anatomy and Physiology of Farm Animals. Lea and Febiger, 1969.

Ganong, W. F. Review of Medical Physiology. Lange Medical Publications, 4th edition, 1970.

Horrobin, D. F. Medical Physiology and Biochemistry. Edward Arnold, 1968.

Hungate, R. E. The Rumen and its Microbes. Academic Press, 1966, chapters 4, 6 and 7.

Swenson, M. J. (editor). Dukes' Physiology of Domestic Animals. Cornell University Press, 1970.

Index

188   INDEX

Cow (*cont.*)
spermatozoa 151, 156
'summer sterility' 37
thermoneutral zone 180
tubular function 139
vitamin A deficiency 63
vitamin D 64
vitamin K blocking 111
zebu cattle 115, 180
Cranial nerve 12, 15
Cranial pillar 82, 83
Crazy chick disease 65
Creatinine 20
Cretinism 37
Crop fertilization 57
Crypts of Lieberkuhn 77, 78
Cud 83
Cumulus oophoricus (germ hill) 153
Cysteine 53
Cytochrome oxidase 61
Cytoplasm 2, 3, 99, 101, 145

Daily milk production 167, 168, 180
Dalton's law (gas) 133
Dam (foetus) 158–161
Decarboxylation 65, 103
Deficiency
ADH 34
calcium 59
cobalt 62
copper 61, 109
essential amino acids 53, 54
iodine 37
iron 61, 109
magnesium 60
minerals 56
niacin 66
pantothenic acid 66
phosphorus 59
potassium 57
STH 31
sodium 57
thyroid hormone 31, 37
vitamins 62, 65–67, 109
7-Dehydrocholesterol 63
Dendrite (nerve) 10, 11
Deoxyribonucleic acid (DNA) 1, 2, 151
Depolarization 14, 17, 22
Depolymerizing enzymes 89
Deposition
bone calcium 39

calcium 64
fat 50
phosphorus 64
protein 50
Derived lipids 55
Derived protein 53
Dermatitis 66
Deutrium oxide 3
Dextrins 52, 75
Diabetes insipidus 34, 143
Diabetes mellitus 44, 45
Diaphragm 126, 129, 130
Diarrhoea 85
Diastolic period 121, 125
Dicoumarol 65, 111
Diffusion 4–6, 69, 96, 134, 162
non-diffusible ions 6
Digestion 50, 51
cellulose 80, 88, 89, 91
enzymes 75
micro-organisms 65
protein 73
proteolytic 93
starch 73, 74
Diglyceride 54, 78
Dioestrus 154, 155
Dipeptidase 75
Diploid chromosome number 157
Direct calorimetry 174
Disaccharides 51, 52, 74, 90, 171
Dissociation curve (oxy-haemo-globin) 134, 135
Distal portion of nephron (kidney) 34
Distal tubule 138, 143
Distension of bladder 144
Dog, stomach, function of 70ff
Donnan equilibrium 5, 139
Donor blood 113, 114
Drinking 68
Ducts
alveolar 128
bile 74, 77, 108
mammary 167, 168
renal 137
Duodenum 71–74, 76–78
Dura 28
Dwarfing 37

Ear 25–27
Effective osmotic pressure 5
Efferent nervous system 12, 14, 29, 71, 132
Eggshell 63, 64